PATIENTOLOGY

PATIENTOLOGY

Toward the Study of Patients

Pamela J. Brink RN PhD FAAN

Copyright @ 2017 Pamela J. Brink RN PhD FAAN
All rights reserved.
ISBN: 1541191064
ISBN 13: 9781541191068
Library of Congress Control Number: 2016921196
CreateSpace Independent Publishing Platform
North Charleston, South Carolina

Also by Pamela J. Brink

Pamela J. Brink, Robert A. Brink, John W. Brink. 2016. *Only by the Grace of God: One Family's Story of Survival during World War II as Prisoners of War in the Philippines.* Bloomington, IN: Archway Publishing

Brink, Pamela J. Ed. 1976. *Transcultural Nursing: A Book of Readings.* Upper Saddle River, New Jersey: Prentice-Hall. Reissued by Waveland Press, Inc. Long Grove, Il. 1990.

Brink, Pamela J. and Marilynn J. Wood. 1988. *Basic Steps in Planning Nursing Research: From Question to Proposal.* Sudbury, MA: Jones & Bartlett, Publishers.

Brink, Pamela J. and Marilynn J. Wood. 1998. *Advanced Design in Nursing Research.* Thousand Oaks, CA: Sage Publications.

CONTENTS

Preface		ix
Acknowledgment		xv
Chapter 1	What Is Patientology?	1
Chapter 2	Patients Are Not Alike: Systems of Classification	10
Chapter 3	The Patient's Place in the Health-Care Delivery System	16
Chapter 4	The Patient's Career: On Moving through the System	26
Chapter 5	The Patient as a Victim	41
Chapter 6	The Patient's Perspective	60
Chapter 7	A Final Note: Toward a Science of Patientology	69
References		75
About the Author		79

PREFACE

When I started to write this book in 1974, I was an assistant professor of nursing at UCLA, with a joint appointment in the department of anthropology. My academic training as a psychiatric nurse and a cultural anthropologist led me to try blending the two fields. I was on my first sabbatical leave, waiting for a travel visa to Nigeria to begin my research on health-care decision-making in a rural Annang community. Since the villagers had three different sources for health care, how did they decide which to use? The visa did not come through until October. In the meantime, I had to have something to show for a year's leave.

That summer I read a book in the field of criminology called *Victimology* (Schafer 1968), which described the scientific study of the victims of crimes. I was struck by several parallels between what the author said about the victims of crimes and what I had seen of the treatment of several of my friends who had had bad experiences at hospitals. Elderly friends in nursing homes were scolded and neglected by the staff. Physicians made diagnoses and gave pronouncements about what the patient was to do without making sure the patient understood the diagnosis or treatment regimen. Gays and lesbians who had been living together for years were not allowed to visit their partners in critical care because they were not "family," even though there was no other family living nearby. The patient's wishes were ignored.

One woman, dying of cancer, asked that she not be given her pain medication on the days her son visited. She wanted to be awake and alert for his visits and not comatose from the medication. The ward nursing staff agreed and did not give her the medication. Her physician was furious! The nurses had no right to countermand his orders. The nursing supervisor was called in to give the medication, and the woman slept through her son's visit. They never had a chance to say good-bye to each other before she died. This was an example of the callousness and disregard for the patient's wishes I have observed.

I attended a one-week invitational course in Washington, DC, on medical ethics a few years later. I was the chair of the ethics-review committee at the UCLA School of Nursing, so this was an opportunity to learn the similarities and differences in research protocols across health disciplines. Examples of the unethical behaviors of health professionals, especially in their research, were provided. One example was using male prisoners in an experimental treatment program for syphilis. Prisoners were included in this experiment without their knowledge, not having been asked for their consent to be research subjects nor told what the research entailed. As is usual in clinical medical research, there was always one group who received no treatment at all. The placebo group, of course, progressed to stage-three syphilis.

This seminar was the first time I realized just how much patients were ignored or disregarded in our health-care delivery system (HCDS). One gut-wrenching story was of an unwanted newborn the mother did not want given up for adoption. (This was in the days before abortion was legalized.) The baby was placed in a bassinette and put in an out-of-the-way place on the ward. She was left alone to starve to death, and the nursing staff had to hear her crying all day long. It took her longer to die than expected because some nurses could not stand it and fed her, thereby prolonging her suffering. I was appalled at the story. The treatment of the baby was inhumane, as if she were not a person in her own right.

So while I was stuck at home waiting for my visa to arrive, I remembered the *Victimology* book and wondered what would be the best way to call attention to what I considered serious unprofessional behavior. Most health professionals are completely unaware they run roughshod over their patient's feelings or desires. Some are not interested in the patient's point of view. They are more concerned with the task than the person.

My concern eventually blossomed into the idea that the study of patients as patients could be given status by a catchy title both as a reference point and for its shock value. So I came up with the term "Patientology." Whenever I have casually mentioned Patientology, people have looked startled, asked what it meant, and eventually become hooked on the idea.

At the time, nursing professionals were struggling with becoming independent practitioners. Nurses felt their relationship with patients was a contractual one and insisted that patients be referred to as "clients." Writing a book about "patients" was considered old-fashioned. Perhaps the climate for a book called *Patientology* is more favorable now.

When I discussed the idea of a Patientology book with my academic superiors, those who would decide my career as an academic, they told me not to bother as "it had already been done. Don't waste your time." Today, I no longer need to worry about pleasing my superiors to achieve promotion and tenure. I can please myself. This book idea has been bothering me for years. It is time to get it off my to-do list.

Although I was discouraged from publishing the book, I did publish an article in *Nursing Outlook* called "Patientology: Just Another Ology?" in 1978. In 1984, I decided to see if the idea of Patientology held any interest for nurses, especially the notion of the patient as a victim of the HCDS, and published "The Patient as Victim." In 1991, hoping they would stir up some interest in the idea, I wrote two editorials for the *Western Journal of Nursing Research*. The first was "Patientology One More Time," and the second was "When Patientology Is Ignored: The Case of Nazi Germany."

I thought these publications had fallen on deaf ears, but this year, when I decided to finish the book, I did a Google search on "Patientology." I was surprised and pleased to see recent articles and a PhD dissertation (Ludvigsen 2009) with "Patientology" in their titles. My article "The Patient Role" (1985) and another article on patient-centered care explore additional aspects of Patientology. Hoyle (1980) suggested that Patientology be a special focus in family medicine which he re-iterated later (Hoyle 1981).

There are currently many articles and books about patients in all health-science fields, based either on research or personal experience. The problem is in accessing them. It's hard to find a specific patient-centered discussion through an Internet search. An umbrella concept could bring together all these disparate sources and topics under one heading: "Patientology."

This book is not intended as a definitive treatise on the study of patients. Instead, it is an outline of some of the areas of study I believe fall under this title. There has been research in some areas, especially in medical sociology and nursing, but there is no consistent niche where these studies can be grouped. I wrote this book to be a catalyst for discussion, research, and further delineation. To that end, each chapter in this book covers an idea fragment but is not exhaustive.

Articles dealing with patient-centered care focus on staff education, suggesting ways in which staff can be less self-focused and more attentive to the patients' needs. These articles are an attempt to change staff attitudes toward patients without admitting or acknowledging that patients are being victimized by staff attitudes (Mayerson 1976).

Patients are pivotal to the HCDS, yet they are frequently ignored. In fact, patients don't appear in organizational charts; they are merely assumed to exist.

Patients have a right to a science of their own. A label denoting a field of study about patients could raise their status. Patients, as a group, have been neglected in comparison to the studies on health professionals and pathologies. I am delighted to see that VIA University College has recently initiated a new program in nursing called "Program for Research and Innovation in Patientology," headed by Anita Haahr, PhD. I look forward to seeing the results of their work in Patientology.

This book is not updated. It is the original concept about how a study of patients could be organized. It is written for anyone who believes, as I do, that the patient is an integral part of the health system. I hope it will interest health professionals and their students, social scientists and their students, administrators, and potential patients.

ACKNOWLEDGMENT

My thanks to Joan Liebmann-Smith, PhD, who was the developmental editor for this manuscript. She was a companion in my thinking, corrected my mistakes, and suggested different ways of expressing my ideas. I am deeply grateful.

CHAPTER 1
WHAT IS PATIENTOLOGY?

"Patientology" means the study of patients. Whenever "-ology" is attached to a word, it means the study of that topic. Most sciences use "-ology" in the names of their specialty fields; for example, cardiology is the study of the heart, anthropology is the study of *anthrōpos* or humans, and bacteriology is the study of bacteria. You get the picture. In the same way, "Patientology" refers to the specific study of patients.

Most people want to be pain free, to be as comfortable as possible while ill, to be cared for when they cannot care for themselves. In addition, they want intelligent, knowledgeable, expert care.

The health sciences—all of them—have focused on the diagnosis, prevention, treatment, cure, and care of illnesses and injuries. This is as it should be. Concomitantly, the health professions have developed the cult of efficiency. In their desire to provide the most effective and efficient services, they have forgotten that it was people, and not diseases, who were receiving this highly specialized technical service. The patient, the owner of the disease, was lost in the rush to tend to the pathology.

"Patient" is the word used to label people (and animals) who are the recipients of some form of health-care services. Patients come in all shapes and sizes, ages, cultures, religions, races, genders, and health statuses. Patients can enter the health-care system voluntarily or involuntarily and leave the system with or without medical advice or help. Patients can be long-term or short-term, legitimate or illegitimate, inpatient or outpatient. Patients can have all kinds of diseases, disabilities, and genetic issues needing a wide variety of health-care solutions. In addition, patients may seek out a variety of health-care providers.

Why Study Patients?
Why should we study patients? Without patients, there would be no health-care delivery system (HCDS). Yet the patient is frequently overlooked by the health system in its attempt to increase the efficiency of its service. In organizational charts of hospitals or community health centers, the patient is not acknowledged. Patients are assumed to exist.

There are as many definitions of patients as there are health professionals and social scientists. The primary concept of the patient, however, is that of the individual who needs and receives the services of the health-care delivery system. Every individual is a potential or actual patient at some time in his or her life needing preventive or healing services. Nevertheless, a person does not become a patient without entering the health-care system for services.

Patients are not alike. They differ demographically as well as in their pathologies, reactions to illnesses, health histories, beliefs about the causes and treatments of illnesses, and senses of responsibility for their own health care. Health professionals treat patients differently according to their pathology, length of time in the system, perception of the patient's needs, perception of the patient's degree of responsibility for causing the condition, and the patient's place in the social system.

This book examines the concept of the patient from many of these aspects as well as the patient role and the patient as a victim. Part of this book parallels the ideas found in the book *Victimology*.

Studying how patients choose their providers and move through the health-care system (Chapman 1975), how they handle their diagnoses, how well they comply with recommended treatments, how they view the system and its personnel, and how they tolerate and live with their symptoms are all part of Patientology.

There are many studies of patients and their perspectives (McGovern 1973), including studies of the patients' role in the hospital (Greenblatt 1957), their role in the education of health professionals, and the degree of their engagement with care. Patient-centered care (Hopkins 1972) and patient advocacy are as much a part of Patientology as the patient role and the sick role.

"Patientology" is a convenient descriptive title under which all these studies would fall. One day, perhaps, there might even be a *Journal of Patientology*!

There are many ways to study patients. If all these studies could be grouped under one umbrella, they would be easier to find, gaps in knowledge could be identified, and comparable studies could be more easily grouped. Researchers in the fields of medical sociology, medical anthropology, and medical economics (Bates 1968) have published many patient-centered articles that are unknown to one another. In general, health professionals do not read one another's literature. Medicine (especially family medicine), nursing (Chirco 1963), chiropractic, dentistry, nutrition/dietetics, pharmacy, laboratories, and clinical pastoral care all publish patient-centered articles that are generally unnoticed by other disciplines. Yet the patient moves from one health discipline to the other daily. When there is little to no sharing of information across these disciplines, the patient is the one who suffers.

Patientology can and should crosscut all disciplines that offer some form of health care or health information. Folk medicine is as important to study as Christian Science (Hoffman 1958) or faith healing. Studies of patients can be qualitative or quantitative. Personal stories (Abramson 1956) can be as valuable as a clinical trial. There are numerous ways to study patients. So long as they use valid forms of data collection and follow ethical standards (Ramsey 1970), they should all offer valuable information.

What Can We Learn from the Study of Patients?
There is a variety of issues that warrant study. It is the patient who receives health-care services, but how does the patient feel about the process and the outcome? Do the patient's feelings impact the decision to stay in the system? Will the patient comply with or fight the health provider? Does it depend on the patient's culture or personality or the way he or she sees the provider or system? Is this even important to the health-care provider or system? With whom does the patient interact while receiving services? Is the patient treated as someone who can understand and cooperate, or is the patient treated as the recipient of commands? How is the patient expected to behave, and who teaches the patient appropriate behavior?

The patient is not just a single individual. The patient is also an espoused couple, a family, or an entire community. The patient can even be a nation. Since health care is not delivered to individuals alone, the same questions asked about the individual can be asked of larger groups.

When the patient is an entire community, to what extent does the political system influence health care? Governments, whether local or national, are expected to be concerned with the health and welfare of its citizens. Whether spraying for mosquito control, ensuring sanitation services such as garbage collection and removal of toilet waste, or providing clean water, local governments are intimately involved in preventing disease in their communities. To what extent are they patient oriented, monitoring their processes to ensure quality service? Who is held responsible if they fail?

While patients are the recipients of some form of health service, the service is not always provided by a designated health professional, especially in the case of preventive health services. Local, state, and national governments are also involved in preventive health services.

To what extent does the educational system influence the health of citizens? Are children taught basic hygiene in schools? Are the food services and waste services in schools directed toward disease prevention? Are playgrounds safe places for children to play without being hurt? What about programs for the prevention of communicable diseases in schools? To what extent are the children and their families involved in the decision-making? Drug abuse is currently a major health issue; to what extent do health-education institutions try to counteract this trend?

Health education is not limited to schools and health-care facilities; the news and entertainment industries are also involved. What is their responsibility for providing accurate information? Drug abuse appears to be common among entertainers and athletes. These individuals are role models for children who try to emulate them. If their heroes do drugs, they are at increased risk of doing so as well.

The above examples fall under the public health system. Because people are affected by the public health system in one way or another, they are its patients. To what extent are the patients' needs and wants considered in these situations? If drug abuse is a major health problem, what is the public health system doing about it? What provisions for inpatient detoxification or rehabilitation centers are provided by the community? What about self-help groups such as Alcoholics Anonymous or Drug Addicts Anonymous?

Every five years, the federal government issues guidelines on what is considered a healthy diet for Americans. To what extent are these guidelines influenced by self-interested groups rather than valid research findings? Health agencies and citizens are expected to comply with these guidelines, but what has been the impact of these guidelines on citizens over the years? Does a one-size-fits-all guideline meet everyone's needs? How do people live and eat within these guidelines?

There seems to be a disconnect between education about healthy eating and the media that advertises unhealthy eating. Television ads promote sweet and sugary drinks, high-fat and high-carbohydrate fast foods, cookies, chips, and candy. Every ad tells children and their parents how good these foods are and how much fun it is to eat them. Yet these ads directly contradict the national guidelines for healthy eating. For the average citizen to comply with government guidelines while being bombarded with enticing foods is impossible. Overconsumption of these foods is said to be the basis of the obesity epidemic, and it is the patient who is blamed for becoming obese. In the end, it is the patient who loses.

In all these matters, to what extent does the patient have a say in the decision-making process? If anything goes wrong, to whom does the patient turn for help? What do citizens do when muddy water comes out of their taps or when lead levels in the water are too high? What do citizens do when these problems continue for years?

Where do citizens fit within these frameworks? Patients are not organized into unions, so their voices have no real clout. Their pleas for help are often ignored in favor of self-interest by the local government, health-professional organizations, or other stakeholders. In the United States, as I suspect in most Western cultures, money talks. The person or group with the most money usually has the most influence, the most political clout. Patients who don't have financial backing, don't speak the language, and don't belong to pressure groups are at a disadvantage, and their voices are not heard. It is up to the health-care system to make the voices of patients heard.

These questions and issues belong in the field of Patientology. It is the patient's welfare and concerns that are so frequently ignored by both health professionals and government officials. When the patient is ignored, in any environment, it is the patient who suffers, not the provider of services (P. Brink, 1991).

Meeting patients' needs is an area in which the health-care delivery system (HCDS) believes itself to be expert. Dieticians and nutritionists are hired to meet the patient's nutritional needs, yet patients often refuse to eat hospital food because it's unappetizing. Nurses are hired to provide care needs, yet patients may refuse medications, treatments, or basic hygiene measures. The physician provides a diagnosis and a treatment plan, yet the patient may reject both. Is the patient responding to the definition of the need for a medical cure or the way in which the problem and its solution are presented?

If the HCDS is the only legitimate source for prevention, diagnosis, treatment, and care of patients, why is it some people seek out alternative methods of health-care delivery or none?

Understanding the Whole Patient
Each patient is unique. Whether the patient is an individual, family, or community, health-care needs are influenced by genetics, personality, culture, and history.

The study of lives—anyone's life—is a fascinating journey into the unknown. Exploring the histories of people's lives in prison, in bars, and in concentration camps reveals strengths and weaknesses, philosophers and scamps, the human and the divine. Studying patients' lives is as fascinating and revealing as the study of any other human experience.

Patients are whole human beings in every aspect of living (Robinson 1939). Health professionals see only a small slice of a person's life. Being patients is not all that people are. They are spouses, siblings, children, and parents. They are educated, wealthy, poor, intelligent, or mentally handicapped. When a patient presents to the health professional, all these aspects of themselves come with them; they are not left outside the examining-room door.

Being a patient is usually one small facet of the human experience, a breath in a life space. The experience of being a patient can be disruptive to one's entire life or can be inconsequential. It can be uplifting or demeaning. Being a patient has many meanings.

This is where the Patientologist comes in.

The following is a good description of a Patientologist. The wife of my chiropractor, a friend of mine, shared what he said in answer to colleagues who were complaining that their patients were not following instructions.

> You first must figure out where the patient is with their condition or whatever the issue is, what their belief system is about, where they are at, what they want to do about it, or if there is anything they want to do about it. If you start with their view and what they want from a treatment, you can then start giving them other big-picture ideas that they may come back to when they are ready. One step at a time in the order that makes sense to them. It's their life, their body. If they want to smoke, not exercise, et cetera…start with where they are at. If they are respected and get results that please them, they are more likely to ask for more later. Some people say they want you to just do what you think is best, but when given two options, they will then choose one. It's always first 'do no harm,' and not respecting a patient is harmful. Do you want to be a doctor, a healer, or a technician? We have too many technicians. We are not machines. We need doctors.

Patientology should become part of the systematic study of all aspects of the health system. Patientology would lead to research, theory, and education about patients as an integral part of health-professional services. Patientology would then become part of the core of who health professionals are and inevitably make them better at caring for their patients.

CHAPTER 2

PATIENTS ARE NOT ALIKE: SYSTEMS OF CLASSIFICATION

For a science of Patientology to exist, having a system for classifying patients into different categories is essential. There are several possible classification systems because patients differ from one another on several dimensions. Currently, most classifications involve the type of service provided, which depends on pathology, acuteness (Jones 1973), settings, and the demographic characteristics of the patient. Other systems of categorization, which may or may not be generally acknowledged, include the legitimacy of the patients' claim for services, the degree to which patients caused their own problems, and decisions about care based on the patients' behaviors. For example, behavioral problems are generally treated in psychiatric settings rather than in general hospitals.

Categorizing and labeling patients by the services provided is obvious and easy but not comprehensive. There are other key variables to consider. For example, patient labels can be explicit (the cancer patient, the broken arm, the outpatient) or not (the compliant patient, the difficult patient, the destructive patient). Making covert labels (such as the complaining patient and the noncompliant or uncooperative patient) (McGregor, 1967) overt may reveal the tensions between staff and patients that could affect treatment and care outcomes.

The following categories are not exhaustive; they are simply suggestions of useful categories for classifying patients.

Classification by Pathology
Because the health-care delivery system (HCDS) is highly specialized, it is more efficient to organize services around pathologies. The patient, then, becomes known by the pathology: the cancer patient, the orthopedic patient, the alcoholic, the new mom, the psychotic patient, the suicide.

Classification of patients by pathology dictates what types of services will be needed for care or cure. A cancer diagnosis will require distinctly different services and often distinctly different inpatient facilities from those provided to the person diagnosed with Alzheimer's disease.

Classification by Type of "-vention" Service
Health-care delivery services are generally dictated not only by the type of pathology (cancer, mental illness, communicable disease) but by the type of service provided (medicine, surgery, emergency care) and whether the service provided will be for acute or chronic care. The type of service can also be dictated by age (pediatrics), gender (OB/GYN), and ability to pay. (At one time, Catholic hospitals had an indigent ward for those unable to pay for their hospitalization and its services.)

The type of "-vention" service provided for any of the above categories will dictate how the patient will be treated and how the patient will respond. Depending on whether the service is prevention (public health), intervention (treatment of the illness/injury in both inpatient and outpatient facilities), or postvention (rehabilitation or recovery from treatment or pathology in both inpatient and outpatient facilities), the patient will have greater or lesser say in the treatment options. (See chapter 3.)

Classification by Demographic Characteristics
Patient age is a major category for organizing services: newborn nursery, pediatric, adult, elderly. In each case the services, personnel, and housing are all dictated simply by the age of the patient. Patients can also be classified by their gender, race, culture, immigrant/refugee status, religion, immigrant nationality, language facility, and education. Health services, however, are not typically dictated by these characteristics.

Classification by Triage Assessment
The concept of triage is usually attached to military field hospitals and emergency rooms. Triage implies an emergency in which a group of people in need of care is brought to a hospital at the same time. Triage determines who needs immediate care versus who can wait. The acuteness of a patient's health problem takes precedence over other patients' inconvenience of having to wait in line. Not only are the acutely ill patients seen first, but they also command a larger number of professionals involved in their service. The same principle holds for postsurgical recovery wards where the most severely ill patients command the greatest attention.

Classification by Voluntariness
People can seek health-care services voluntarily or involuntarily. They can walk into a health-care facility and request services either because they have decided they need professional help or because they have been referred by a health-care provider. In contrast, the involuntary patient may have no choice. For example, victims of automobile accidents can be brought to the emergency room by ambulance services or by family members. They may not even be

conscious. Alcoholics, addicts, and anorexics may also be involuntary admissions into a health-care facility.

The interaction between patients and staff can be colored by voluntariness. Involuntary patients may or may not be cooperative. They may fight the admission, especially if they belong to a religious group that does not believe in Western medicine or if they are in denial about their illness.

Classification by Length of Care

Not only are health-care services organized around pathologies, but they are organized around the concept of longevity. Inpatient facilities are frequently organized around length of care. Patients are admitted either for acute or chronic care. Thus, patients are involved in the decision-making about health care. Hospitals can be for acute care or for warehousing the elderly with chronic or debilitating ailments. Patients admitted to nursing homes are rarely discharged. On the other hand, patients admitted to rehabilitation facilities are expected to have an eventual discharge home.

Classification by the Legitimacy of the Illness or Injury

Legitimacy is an unacknowledged system of classification. Healthcare providers judge patients based on a loose set of assumptions about whether they deserve health care. Legitimate patients are worthy, whereas illegitimate patients are not.

The characteristics of a legitimate patient are as follows: 1) has no responsibility for the causation of the illness or injury, 2) has a known health problem, 3) is under the care of a legitimate healthcare provider or is in a hospital receiving services, and 4) is compliant with the prescribed treatment plan.

On the other hand, an illegitimate patient 1) has no known pathology, 2) may have deliberately caused the condition, 3) is insistent on medical care despite the lack of a diagnosis, and/or 4) may have a condition that is socially devalued or considered immoral.

In the same way that the patient is considered legitimate/illegitimate, the illnesses with which they present may be as well.

A legitimate illness 1) is one that is well studied and has a diagnosis and/or known symptoms or 2) has symptoms that are so severe they need tending to immediately, whether the cause is known or not, and 3) responds positively to known treatment regimens.

An illegitimate illness, as defined by local or state agencies, 1) has an illegal cause, 2) is being treated by a faith healer or "quack," 3) is a communicable disease that was not reported, and/or 4) has symptoms that are believed to be manufactured by the person seeking services.

Classification by a Patient's Degree of Responsibility for the Health Problem
A lesser-known system of categorization is the staff's or provider's decision about the patient's degree of responsibility for disease causation. (See chapter 6). In most cases, both the staff and patient are unaware of this system of classification, which parallels victim typology.

Classification by the Patient's Social Status
Classifying patients by social status does not appear in textbooks. Certain people are considered more "equal" and deserving than others and will always go to the head of a waiting line. Politicians, movie and TV stars, and famous athletes all receive privileged care. They are often treated as if they were royalty. Not only do they go to the head of the line, but their housing and meals are of a higher quality than those of the other patients in an inpatient facility. Generally, they are given private rooms rather than being placed in a four-bed ward housing both men and women. In fact, American politicians have their own higher-quality, completely funded health-care system.

Classification by Patient Behavior

Not all methods of categorizing patients appear on organizational charts. Inpatients are categorized by staff according to their perceived behaviors. Staff prefer compliant patients who cooperate with their care and give them no trouble. The aggressive patient, regardless of whether the behavior is a personality trait or the effect of a stroke, is avoided by staff and is in danger of neglect. These and other troublesome patients can be described as uncooperative, manipulative, hostile, combative, malingering, dependent, and deviant and may be treated or mistreated according to these labels.

Research on patients can be focused on these systems of categorization, or new categories might emerge that merit consideration and study. These old and new categories can dictate where the patient will receive services, how long the service will last, how the patient will be treated by staff, and the degree to which the patient can participate in decision-making regarding services. These classifications influence one another. The importance of their impact on the patient experience is demonstrated throughout this book.

CHAPTER 3

THE PATIENT'S PLACE IN THE HEALTH-CARE DELIVERY SYSTEM

The impression that the patient has a place in the health-care delivery system (HCDS) is incorrect. The patient is not mentioned in any organizational chart of the current HCDS. A Google search of hospital organizational charts does not show patients anywhere. The charts are all about the services provided and how they relate to one another. Health-care delivery refers to the *delivery* of goods and services. The delivery of these services—how they are delivered, who delivers them, how often and in what form they are delivered—are all part of the structure of the HCDS. The patient is the *recipient* of services, not a provider.

The structure of health-care delivery involves the organization of people and services into a hierarchical system of positions, roles, values, and beliefs about delivery. The HCDS is in complete control of all legitimate/legal health-care delivery services. The patient is faced with a monopoly, i.e., a dictatorship, to which he or she must apply for services. (See Greenblatt et al 1957.) The patient assumes the care will be provided according to high ethical and professional standards. In return for these services, the patient is expected to trust the system. These services, as we shall see, may, in fact, fall short of these high standards.

Although the patient has no role in the organizational structure, the patient has an integral part in the functioning of the system.

Patients are the reason for the existence of the HCDS. Patients are the source of revenue that finances the system; they provide the funds needed, whether through direct payments, insurance, government subsidies, or charitable donations. Without patients, there would be no revenue, and there would be no system for health-care delivery.

Another function of patients within an HCDS is as subjects for research or for educating health-profession students. Whether alive or dead, patients serve as guinea pigs for student education. The patient is not always informed that the care provider is a student and has no choice of accepting or rejecting the student. The system makes this decision for the patient.

Patients are absolutely necessary as research subjects. At one time, before the requirement of medical ethics boards, the patient was not always informed of the research project or its risks. Although this has changed, the ethical and professional conduct of health-care research is still under the control of the HCDS and its educational institutions.

Patient/Institution/Provider Contract

Whenever a patient—whether an individual, a family, or a community—interacts with the HCDS, the patient is contracting for services from the system (A. W. Burgess 1976). The interaction is a contract whether either party is aware of it or if it is unwritten. The contractual arrangement will differ depending on the type of services the patient is receiving.

The physician-patient interaction (or healer-patient) is the basic contractual dyad within the HCDS (Cartwright 1967). The potential patient usually seeks out the services of a single healer (physician, nurse, dentist, chiropractor, therapist, clinic, hospital, *curandero*), requests services, and is either accepted or denied services. When the person requesting services is accepted, this constitutes a contract for services to be provided and paid for. The contract, which is unwritten, like the one between a private-business owner and customer, is in the simple two-party agreement for receiving goods and services in exchange for payment of a fee. Both parties agree to the terms.

The difference between the healer-patient contract and the customer–business owner contract is that the fee for service may or may not be agreed to or understood at the time the service is rendered. The patient is not always informed of the degree of responsibility for payment if an insurance company or Medicare is billed first. The patient learns later what is owed.

Type of Health Service Provided

HCDS services are organized around the type of service provided: prevention (preventing illnesses and accidents), intervention (the curing and care process), and postvention (aftercare from surgery or other medical care). Each of these areas does research and evaluation on the services provided. The patient's role as the receiver of services differs in response to the type of service provided.

Prevention Services

Preventive services generally occur in community settings rather than in hospitals. Most Americans are familiar with public health clinics where travel immunizations, inoculations, and well-baby services are provided. In recent times, major grocery chains have begun offering flu shots as well as blood pressure monitors and pharmacy services. Visits to private physicians or community clinics for an annual physical exam, hearing tests, eye exams, or to obtain requisitions for laboratory tests are preventive services. Visits to dentists include dental hygiene as well as oral evaluations with X-rays. A chiropractor will do a physical assessment, including an evaluation of needs. These dentist and chiropractor visits are both screening services as well as short-term check-ups designed to prevent future health problems. Patients may visit regularly for treatment of an ongoing problem or to have an annual "tune-up."

Whether the patient enters the system for crises intervention or prenatal services, these are considered preventive services. The patient is in and out quickly, visits are short, and the intervention is brief. School health programs, educational programs, and eye exams all fall within the area of prevention.

Often, the patient is not ill. There is no physical disability or injury requiring an intervention. The patient decides on the service needed, seeks out the service, then goes home to engage in other activities.

In some cases, preventive services can be coercive—something in which citizens have no choice. Children cannot attend school without having had childhood immunizations. International travelers may not be able to leave the country or return without immunizations. The public-health department may institute fluoridation of water without consulting citizens. Garbage collection and sewage disposal are also preventive services. Eliminating common drinking cups and forbidding spitting on the sidewalk were instituted by the public health department to prevent the spread of tuberculosis. The elimination of lead in water, paint, and gasoline is preventive-health community intervention. Smog control to prevent lung cancer is also a preventive-health public-health initiative. In all these cases, local or national governments have decided that disease prevention is more important than giving the citizen the choice to accept.

In preventive settings, patients are usually in control of their own health care. They may refuse to see health professionals, walk out of clinics, or even choose their providers. The person seeking these services may be referred to as a client rather than as a patient to denote a responsible adult capable of self-determination, self-care, and payment of services.

Sometimes patients go to intervention settings for preventive services. X-rays, lab work, or other diagnostic workup may be available only at the local hospital. In this case, patients receive preventive services in intervention settings. These services may require an overnight stay, which means the patient receives a bed and meals, services normally provided by a hotel. The setting in which services are rendered, as we have seen, dictates the role patients are expected to play. (See chapter 4)

Intervention Services

Most intervention services are provided in inpatient settings. In fact, the label "patient" was coined to denote the person receiving intervention services. Here, it is the pathology that determines the type and length of services the patient will receive. Hospitals are organized around specific pathologies. There are medical wards, surgical wards, orthopedic wards, psychiatric wards, ICUs (intensive care units), emergency services, OB/GYN units, and pediatric units.

Hospitals also include radiology, laboratories, surgical theaters, and sometimes physical therapy. As mentioned above, the hospital offers hotel amenities such as housekeeping, beds, food services, laundry, a business office, grounds keeping, and maintenance. The hospital will also have waiting rooms, some type of cafeteria for families and staff, a gift shop, and perhaps a chapel.

Some intervention services are offered in the provider's office. Dental interventions to treat cavities and periodontal disease are usually performed in a dental office rather than in a hospital. Abortions are a surgical procedure called dilatation and curettage (D&C) but are not normally conducted in a hospital setting. Instead, they are provided in outpatient clinic settings.

Like it or not, patients are known by their pathologies. Pathology is the critical issue in the type and extent of service the patient will receive. Hospitals are organized around pathologies. Even the smallest hospital will have a maternity ward separated from all other treatment facilities. Since childbirth is a natural process, maternity wards are essentially preventive services, despite attempts to 'medicalize' birth. If anything goes wrong during labor and delivery, there are professionals and equipment readily available for emergencies.

Not all hospitals will have a psychiatric ward, but if they do, they too are isolated from other patient wards. Psychiatric patients are not physically ill; they have mental issues that can make them unpredictable, perhaps violent or self-destructive, immobilized, or prone to act in other abnormal ways. Some are noisy, combative, or not in control of their bodily functions. They may talk in odd ways or not talk at all. Although these patients are rarely a threat to themselves or others, the public fears them and does not understand them. They want them "put away" where they will not be seen or heard.

The greatest concentration of health-care facilities and providers is in intervention services. Medical science is focused on intervention into pathologies; therefore, medical education, research, patient services, and professional staff all fall within this area. Because of this attention to specific pathologies, the person who has the pathology is frequently neglected or ignored. (This is treated chapter 5, "The Patient as a Victim.") The intervention model presupposes the patient is a passive recipient. Staff attitudes often reflect this assumption as well. Once admitted, the patient abandons all decision-making unless granted by the provider. The patient cannot move in or out of the intervention setting at will; the provider's permission is required. For all intents and purposes, once admitted to the facility, the patient belongs to the system.

Postvention Services
The third area patients can be found is in postvention services or aftercare. Whether the patient is discharged home after surgery to be cared for by a paraprofessional or professional nurse—or referred to physical therapy—postvention refers to rehabilitation, convalescence, follow-up services, terminal hospice home care, or other long-term chronic-disease management outside a hospital setting. Depending on the type of postvention services needed, patients need intermittent rather than constant supervision.

Some patients will never be cured; they are either too old or have serious birth defects, terminal illnesses, or chronic illnesses. This is an area that receives the least interest or funding. Since no cure is anticipated, there is no real challenge. The focus becomes care rather than cure.

Summary
The quality of services, the amount of research, and the time devoted to the education of health professionals all reflect the degree of interest in the patients within each of these "-vention" settings. The basic interest in the patient is as a disease-bearing organism.

In preventive settings, the cause of the disease is known, and a treatment program has been developed to prevent the associated problems. Here the patient is treated as a self-motivating customer or client who is contracting for short-term services.

In intervention settings, the disease is known or is being studied, and every attempt is made to achieve a cure. Depending on the pathology and treatment, the patient is acted on and is not considered a partner in the process.

In postvention settings, either the patient recovers normal functioning at home or no cure is anticipated. In the latter case, the patient lives with the health problem. Since the HCDS was devised to postpone death, prevent disease or injury, or cure it, the patient who cannot get well is the least preferred. This patient is a constant reminder of the failure of medical science.

The function, then, that the patient performs for the HCDS is based on the patient being a receiver of services, whether those services are in preventive, interventive, or postventive settings—or a combination of all three. The patient is an indispensable part of the total functioning of the system. There would be no HCDS without patients.

The Patient's Place in the Health System

To place the patient on an equal status with that of health professionals, one of the first steps would be to eliminate the label "health-care delivery system," with all its connotations, and substitute "health system" (Mark Field 1973) instead. "Health culture" has been proposed as another alternative and, in many respects, is an improvement over "health system."

The label "health system" incorporates all facets of health within its social/structural contexts, including patients and their families (or other support systems), health professionals, health education (both public and specialized), health theory and research, delivery services, health agencies, and so on. The emphasis is on health and disease, all social roles involved in health, all bureaucracies directly and indirectly involved, and the relationship between the health system and all other organizational/social systems in society.

The change in emphasis from a delivery system, or even a care system, would have to include the patient as an equal and contributing member of the system. Instead of focusing on the providers of services, the new concept would require an analysis of the contractual relationship between giver and receiver. When only one party to a contract is evaluated, the results of the analysis are distorted. The rights and responsibilities of both parties need to be examined.

The basic and primary contract is between the patient (whether individual, family, or community) and the healer/provider. When intervention services are provided in intervention settings, the contract involves the patient, healer, and hospital. Generally, the contract with the hospital is written to protect the hospital, its providers, and its services. The hospital is responsible for the technical competence of its personnel and equipment as well as for their professional behavior. The hospital is responsible for supervising, screening, and educating its employees for the delivery of safe, ethical, and competent health care. Staff are responsible to the hospital (their employer), not the patient.

Whether the patient is in preventive, interventive, or postventive settings, the nature of the contractual arrangement does not alter measurably. The patient may be contracting for services from a private practitioner (physician or other health-care provider) or a medical corporation (hospital or outpatient facility) at the same time. The contract requires the patient to agree and comply with services prior to being accepted.

Where the label "health-care delivery system" is exclusive, the label "health system" is inclusive, allowing for the patient's beliefs and values, home remedies, and alternative health providers and systems.

To call attention to patients as an integral part of this contract for services, the organizational chart could be relabeled as the "health system" (HS), leaving out the terms "care delivery." The patient, then, becomes an integral part of the health system as the recipient of care. Where patients are only understood to exist in an organizational chart devoted to the structure for the delivery of services, in a Health System, patients are an integral part of the system. Research on patients would have an umbrella framework within which to place these studies.

Instead of being in a one-down position, the patient can become a coparticipant in health, with all the rights and privileges afforded to adults functioning in other systems. Contracts for services will protect the patient as well as the provider and delivery agency, and the patient will have an equal right to be heard.

Unless the focus changes from delivery to health, the patient will continue to be ignored.

CHAPTER 4

THE PATIENT'S CAREER: ON MOVING THROUGH THE SYSTEM

The Potential Patient

Everyone is a potential patient. Sometime between conception and death, every person will have contact with at least one service of the health-care delivery system (HCDS). Whether that contact comes from listening to TV ads for medications, being exposed to the Public Health Service's annual flu-shot drive, seeing a doctor for an annual physical, being taken to the emergency room following an accident, having health screenings while in school or to renew a driver's license, or even being killed while in the womb, everyone will eventually encounter the HCDS. The system is everywhere, whether obvious or obscure, and everyone is subjected to its rules and regulations.

Every American has a stake in the US system of health-care delivery. Every American has the right to monitor the system for its efficiency, competence, ethics, availability, professionalism, and outcomes. Sick people do not have the energy to monitor the system—healthy people do.

The potential patient has the right to choose the HCDS most suited to the health problem as well as the practitioner or institution for services. It is the consumer's responsibility to discover just how competent the practitioner or institution is and how much it will cost. The consumer can choose a *curandero* or faith healer but is responsible for the consequences of that choice.

The Western HCDS remains the primary lawful system for providing health care. Anyone choosing certain unsanctioned alternative services, especially for children, may be arrested. One family was arrested for taking their diabetic son to a faith healer rather than a physician.

The community, as potential patients, can establish consumer groups to monitor the system (Hochbaum 1969). These groups can request periodic monitoring of physicians/healers just as banks have periodic monitoring by accountants. The community can establish a system, like the jury system, in which potential patients and former patients can serve on review boards, accreditation boards, licensing boards, ethics committees, and so on. All too often, citizen committees are composed of prominent citizens, not former patients who were the most likely to suffer from the system.

On Becoming a Patient

Who Makes the Decision to Seek Health Care?

Adults usually make their own decisions whether or not to seek health care, although significant others may encourage or discourage their decisions. Children and the elderly frequently will have the decision made for them. Sometimes it is the health-care system that makes the decision. For instance, when people resist seeking health care for a communicable disease, the health-care system might step in and make the decision for them.

To become a patient, an individual must be accepted into the system by a health professional (physician, dentist, chiropractor). To be legitimized, the potential patient who has self-defined as being ill or in need of preventive services must be brought to the attention of the HCDS, either voluntarily or by the actions of others. Until accepted as a patient by the HCDS, an individual is simply ill, injured, or in need of services.

Routes to Becoming a Patient
As mentioned in chapter 2, there are two major routes for entering the health-care system: voluntarily and involuntarily.

Upon entering the system, the individual is labeled a patient. The voluntary patient is the individual who deliberately seeks out the services of the HCDS; there is no coercion. These are the people who make appointments for services they cannot perform themselves independently, such as eye exams, dental hygiene, chiropractic care, and treatment of extensive burns or cuts that will not stop bleeding. People also seek out doctors for annual physicals or other preventive care and health issues.

The involuntary patient, on the other hand, is brought to the HCDS by others with or without the person's consent. Some are coerced into seeking help. Families or friends may try to get an alcoholic, drug addict, or gambler into a treatment program. A person with a communicable disease is not given much choice about receiving treatment. The mentally ill, who are perceived as being a danger to themselves or others, are often involuntary patients. Jehovah's Witnesses, Christian Scientists, and other similar religious groups may find themselves being coerced into receiving treatments, especially if the patient is a child. An involuntary patient can be a child, an unconscious person, or a victim of an accident or violent crime. An involuntary patient needs care but is either unable or unwilling to seek it.

The Counterfeit Patient
Another type of patient is the spurious or counterfeit patient—the person for whom no diagnosis can be found to explain the symptomology but who keeps coming back. Sometimes a diagnosis is found using newer technologies, but if no diagnosis is found, the patient is suspected of attention-getting. In those cases, the patient may be labelled a malingerer or "crock." The spurious patient is also transient as he or she is admitted and discharged frequently. This patient may also be long-term, continually seeking the system for help throughout life.

To become a patient, therefore, an individual must 1) self-define or be defined by others as needing HCDS services, 2) must be validated by a health professional, and 3) must be provided with the services only the HCDS can provide. Only the HCDS is empowered, by law, to confer and validate the label "patient."

Factors Affecting the Decision-Making Process
The decision to enter the HCDS and become a patient is not usually taken lightly. There are many factors to consider. Dr. Dorrian Sweetser (personal communication) found that among the Boston middle class, the onset, ambiguity, and severity of symptoms were critical to the definition of an illness that would require a physician to diagnose. Symptoms that persist eventually prompt people to seek a cause. Sudden or persistent pain can instigate a doctor's visit. An accident causing excessive bleeding or burns also sends people for help.

Others are hesitant to seek health care. Monetary considerations such as the ability to pay or lack of health-insurance coverage, as well as time off from work, also enter the decision-making process. Some potential patients are afraid their complaints are not "serious enough" to claim a physician's time, while others fear they may be thought of as malingerers if they bring small but uncomfortable symptoms. Some fear the possible diagnosis of cancer or heart disease. Still others believe that if they can continue to function, there is no need to see a physician.

Becoming a patient carries the potential for a disruption of lifestyle, loss of revenue earmarked for other things, and even death. For most people, becoming a patient is a hardship with insufficient rewards to assume the role without a great deal of thought.

Using More Than One HCDS Concurrently

One of the most frustrating findings a health professional can make is that the patient is self-medicating or seeking the services of a folk healer or another type of practitioner. The concern is that the healing methods of the other practitioners, including medications and routines, may conflict with the prescribed treatment. When people combine two or more alternative healing systems, they demonstrate a lack of complete trust in the HCDS healer. The advice of the health professional may be discarded in favor of the advice of the alternative healer.

The one acceptable alternative healing system is religion—so long as it does not completely replace the services of the HCDS. When patients seek a miraculous cure or have prayer circles in conjunction with professional care, these are considered innocuous and perhaps beneficial. On the other hand, anything that contradicts the diagnosis and treatment plan of the HCDS will be frowned upon.

There are times when the HCDS requires the patient to use more than one provider for the same services, which can be a source of frustration and conflict for both the patient and provider.

For example, a Canadian decided to go to Arizona for the winter. She was under the regular care of three dentists in Canada: a general dentist, an orthodontist, and a periodontist. Because she had periodontal disease, she saw a dental hygienist four times a year. Her trip coincided with one of her dental hygiene visits, so she sought out an Arizona dentist to get her teeth cleaned. The dentist told her that he could not provide this service unless he had full mouth X-rays and the results of her most recent periodontal exam. If she could not get these from her Canadian dentists, she would have to pay to have these exams performed in his office. All she wanted was to get her teeth cleaned, but the dentist wanted to treat her as his patient. So, just to get her teeth cleaned this one time, she now had two general dentists, an orthodontist, and a periodontist.

On another visit, she had forgotten to bring the X-rays and periodontal records with her. The dental hygienist insisted on doing a periodontal exam. After she refused and the hygienist began cleaning, she felt the hygienist probing. She stopped her and said, "I asked you not to probe my gums."

The hygienist replied, "I didn't think you would notice."

The Dentistry Dilemma
Dentistry is a good example of how the HCDS fails to take the patient's needs into consideration. In many communities, a medical walk-in clinic will be staffed by physicians, nurse practitioners, and other licensed practitioners qualified to diagnose, treat, and prescribe medications. Patients can walk in for a specific problem; get a diagnosis, referral, prescription, lab work, or X-rays; and leave. The relationship between health-care provider and patient is transient rather than long-term.

Unlike medicine, and except for dental schools, dentistry does not have walk-in clinics for the immediate treatment of specific issues. Dentistry still relies on the small-business model of one (or more) dentists operating a dental office that provides several services. If it is a general practice, the dentist will provide examinations, X-rays, oral surgeries, and dental hygiene. Patients may then be referred to specialty dentists such as orthodontists or periodontists, who will then send a report back to the primary dentist.

Although dentistry has been a leader in prevention research and services for oral health, there are no oral hygiene clinics where patients can get their teeth cleaned on a routine basis. (These clinics would be staffed by dental hygienists and not dentists.) Patients must go to a dentist's office for this service. This poses a problem for patients who travel, as demonstrated above.

Here is the dilemma: The patient wants only a cleaning; the dentist wants to have a complete dental record and oral history. The patient must either submit to, and pay for, X-rays and periodontal exams at each dental office or have these reports faxed before treatment can begin. The question becomes, whose needs are being met?

Perhaps community dental organizations could develop preventive dental services similar to those provided in dental schools.

Dental schools train dental hygienists as well as dentists. The school will offer individuals outpatient clinics for dental hygiene, oral surgeries, gum resections, cavity repairs, or extractions. The dental school does not require a full dental history for these services. It is a transient patient facility created to provide patients for students to use as learning subjects. The clinics are run primarily for the benefit of student learning while also providing care to the indigent patient. The patient can have a dental problem taken care of without having to enter into a full dentist-patient-contract relationship. For many people, having access to this type of transient dental service in their community would be a good thing.

On Being a Patient

Once accepted into the HCDS as a legitimate recipient of healthcare services, the person becomes a patient. At this point, the person has a new role and must learn to behave appropriately in that role.

In 1951, Talcott Parsons introduced the concept of "the sick role" in his book *The Social System*. He described the behaviors expected of persons who are ill. The sick person is exempted from

Patientology

all other social obligations for the entirety of the illness experience and is assumed to need professional assistance to get well. In other words, self-help will not cure the sick person. The person is expected to want to get well. Most sick people want to be cared for, coddled, if you will, while they are feeling miserable. They don't want to have to problem-solve, care for others, or participate in self-care.

People can take on the sick role voluntarily or involuntarily. Taking on the role may be influenced by whether the illness can be cared for at home or is severe enough to require professional help.

But what of people who are not ill but need health services for prevention or other reasons?

Not all patients are sick, although there are points of convergence. Many sick people never seek out the HCDS and, therefore, never become patients. The patient role is a set of behavioral expectations in relation to other roles in the HCDS. The normative patient role is based on being in an inpatient facility. The role shifts and changes when the patient is in an outpatient facility or is simply a potential patient receiving health education or immunizations.

Definition of "Role"

Roles are the behaviors or actions associated with social positions. Every society has expected norms for behavior that are either implicit or explicit. In any social group, people don't know how to respond to one another unless there are rules everyone follows. The rules apply very specifically to each social position. When people act outside these expectations, they are considered deliberately deviant, ignorant, or crazy. Every social system teaches these roles to its members.

There are two different sets of roles everyone learns: roles that are either ascribed or achieved. Everyone is assigned both sets of roles and expected to blend them appropriately. When individuals refuse to act according to their roles, other people have no idea how to respond appropriately.

Ascribed roles are the roles assigned to individuals based on the "accidents" of birth: gender, age, social class, race, and culture. Women are expected to behave differently from men. Although these gender-specific roles are blurring in modern secular societies, certain expectations still exist. In the same sense, there are behaviors associated with a person's calendar age. An adult is not expected to behave as a child behaves. Children are forgiven for behaviors that would not be forgiven in adults. Individuals learn the behaviors expected of them through interactions with others; each is expected to learn acceptable behavior and avoid unacceptable behavior. In most societies, all adults are assumed to have the responsibility of correcting the behaviors of children. No one wants adult deviants in society. Deviants break the rules. Decisions must be made as to what should be done with them.

In contrast, achieved roles are earned. It is not enough just to be a male child; that male child is expected to grow up to be a responsible adult. That doesn't happen simply by getting older. The child is expected to learn the rules and gain the knowledge that will ensure he is a contributing member of society. So children attend classes on subjects considered basic to that society. Mathematics, writing/communication skills, a sense of history, and the social systems that make up the society are all considered basic. These subjects also prepare people for future occupations. Jobs/occupations are achieved through study and/or practice just as athletic achievement takes long hours of practice. These roles are earned through personal, individual effort.

An ascribed role is conferred on an individual and may be (the transgendered person is an individual who rejects the ascribed role associated with genitals) lifelong, whereas an achieved role is not. One is not born a physician or a nurse. Persons must achieve these titles through an educational or training process. Once achieved, however, the title is never taken away, even when the person retires. In some cases, a person's ascribed role will limit the choices available for achieved roles. In many societies, women are denied the education given to men simply because they are women. Most importantly, everyone is expected to behave appropriately according to both ascribed and achieved roles at the same time.

The Patient Role Is an Ascribed Role
"Patiency" (or being a patient) is an ascribed role. Patients are people who have been accepted as valid recipients of health-care services. Whether they seek services voluntarily or involuntarily, they are labeled as patients and expected to understand that they have a definite role to play within the health-care system. Like all other ascribed roles, patients learn how to behave appropriately only through interactions with the members of the HCDS (Katz & Kahn 1964).

Patient Role as Part of a Role Set
Role theory includes the concept of role set. These are roles that interact with both the sick role and patient role. The role set for the sick role involves the family and significant others and may involve a hospital, physician, or pharmacist. The role set for the patient role includes all members of the HCDS. Since it is the HCDS that confers the status of patient (ascribes the patient role), it is the HCDS's responsibility to teach the patient appropriate role behaviors. Every health-care provider, knowingly or not, teaches the patient the appropriate way to behave in the situation.

The patient role is not a singular role but will be altered by other ascribed roles. For example, child patients are not expected to behave in the same way as adult patients and vice versa. If patients are in an outpatient facility, they are expected to behave differently from an inpatient who is ill or in pain. Patients are treated differently and are expected to behave differently whether inpatients, outpatients, sick patients, well patients, geriatric patients, pediatric patients, suicidal patients, alcoholic patients, and so on. In addition, areas of health-care delivery such as surgery or maternity will place different expectations on patient behavior.

Patient classifications based on pathology, type of intervention, age, gender, and length of care will alter the staff's expectation of patient behavior. If the patient does not conform to staff expectations, a covert system of classification will develop: the hypochondriac, the demanding patient, the aggressive patient, and the difficult patient, among others.

To a greater or lesser degree, all patients are expected to want to get well. Even if the diagnosis is terminal, the patient is expected to fight through their disease. Television news media, in particular, will describe a celebrity as "fighting their disease" as if surviving cancer is like a personal battle with the disease. In a sense, personnel do not like patients who give up or do not try to cooperate with the healing process. When the patient has a terminal or chronic condition, health-care staff become frustrated in their desire to heal because they have nothing to offer. They cannot heal or cure. People who have a lethal diagnosis but refuse health care are also frustrating.

Being a patient with an illness suggests to the health professional that the person wants to cooperate with the treatment process. The patient is expected to comply without fuss and without asking too many questions. Patients are not expected to defy the healer or fight the treatment program. Although patients may ask questions about the disease or treatment program, they are not expected to question the judgments of the health-care provider. Providers can become abrupt and turn patients off if they don't have answers to their questions.

Some patient questions are more acceptable than others. For example, "Did my doctor order this medication?" challenges the competence of the nurse to follow orders. Whereas a question such as "Is my doctor coming to see me today?" is acceptable, the following are not: "Are you sure I can't get any more pain medication right now?" "Why are you taking me to PT? My doctor said I did not have to go to physical therapy today." "I am a diabetic. The food tray you brought me is not a diabetic diet! Why can't I have my diabetic diet?" On the other hand, patients are not expected to question the medications ordered by the physician. They are expected to take the medication and not argue about it. In fact, questioning inpatient staff about any aspect of treatment may be perceived as being difficult. Patients are expected to cooperate fully with all procedures whether they understand them or not. In addition to cooperation, another trait highly valued by health-care staff is gratitude. Whether the services were small or large, expressions of gratitude are appreciated. Grateful patients are cared for more rapidly than ungrateful or grumpy patients.

The Subordinate Position of Patients
An inpatient is in a subordinate position in the hospital hierarchy. My article "The Natural Triad in Health Care" (Brink 1972) grew out of a conversation with Dr. Morris Freilich in which he described his analysis of the relationship between the father and the mother's brother in kinship systems (Freilich 1964). The parallels between his analysis of kinship roles and the relationship between the nurse and the physician as opposed to the patient were striking. The physician is at the head of the triad; the nurse or nurse's aide is the physician's partner in providing care; and, as the recipient, the patient is at the bottom of the triad. The patient is expected to understand and accept this arrangement.

This subordinate position also occurs in outpatient settings. A patient with a facial growth was referred to a dermatologist by her dentist. The dermatologist told the patient she, the patient, would receive the pathologist's report on her growth. The patient did not receive the pathologist's report, but her dentist did.

Length of the Patient Role
The HCDS makes the decision on the duration of the patient role. The transient patient is in and out for relatively brief periods and may be either voluntary or involuntary. Immunizations and health-screening services are predominantly for transient patients, who frequently are healthy.

The long-term patient (Minnie. Field 1967) requires attention for an indefinite period; their absolute cure or relief of symptomology is usually in doubt. Genetic anomalies, gerontology, rehabilitation, and hospice all require long-term care. Patients being treated by cardiologists, rheumatologists, chiropractors, and allergists, among others, frequently require long-term care.

Role changes are based on housing and labels. When a patient is transferred from an acute-care inpatient facility to a rehabilitation center, there is a shift in staff expectations for patient behavior. Patients are expected to be more independent, less demanding, and more cooperative with their treatment regimen. When a patient receives the label of "Alzheimer's," "terminal," or "schizophrenic," staff have an entirely different set of behavioral expectations and treat the patient accordingly (French 1973).

On Leaving the System or Terminating the Patient's Career
In general, leaving the system with medical advice refers to being discharged from the hospital or told by the healer that the problem is resolved and no further treatment is necessary. Being discharged with medical advice ensures the patient will be well received if, or when, further medical care is needed.

Another way of being discharged with medical advice is a decision made by the healer that the patient is being uncooperative and not following medical advice. The healer will refuse to see the patient again, believing the patient is not worth the time and effort. Some patients are uncooperative because their perception of the situation is colored by their cultural expectations and experiences (McGregor 1967). Some patients get tired of having surgeries and begin refusing them. The surgeon then discharges the patient as uncooperative. Taking time to discover what is interfering with the treatment plan might benefit both healer and patient.

The patient who discharges him or herself from the hospital or otherwise terminates health-care services either against or without medical advice (AMA) is not welcome to return. That patient is seen as obstinate, ungrateful, or just plain difficult, and no one wants to spread out the welcome mat. Unfortunately, no one examines why that person leaves AMA.

Hanging On
No one wants to spend the rest of his or her life as a patient under the total control of the HCDS. Unfortunately, for many people, some kind of long-term inpatient facility is their destiny, such as chronic care and hospice services for the dying. People with genetic diseases requiring lifelong care, those with mental illnesses, the very elderly, and people with dementia are part of this population. With the aging population and disruption of extended families to care for the disabled elderly, the community must provide housing and care for people who can no longer do so for themselves. Otherwise, they would be homeless and dying in the streets. These patients are subjected to a kind of warehousing. Care is primarily hotel services with basic hygiene thrown in. They have nowhere else to go and no one else to care for them. Some acute-care hospitals find their beds taken up by these patients simply because there is nowhere else to send them.

Patients in these long-term-care service facilities are simply waiting to die. Whether they are still mentally active or have Alzheimer's disease, they have little or no control over their care and may have no family to protect them from abuse or neglect. Stroke survivors, especially men, undergo personality changes. They can be aggressive and have episodes of violent anger, striking out at whomever is around. Staff tend to avoid these patients (Minnie. Field 1967).

Because there is no chance these patients will recover, they tend to be devalued as noncontributing members of society. Community tax dollars are readily spent on patients who will get well again. Long-term-warehousing-care facilities are frequently underfinanced and either understaffed or staffed by ancillary health personnel who may be poorly trained in gerontology.

For these patients, dying is their only way out of the system.

Dying

No health professional likes having patients die while still under treatment or care. Dying is the ultimate failure of the system to cure or heal. The patient may or may not choose to die. Physician-assisted suicide and euthanasia are now becoming legal options ostensibly to give patients the choice to live or die. These legal options also open the door for families or legal guardians to make life-and-death decisions for patients, with or without their consent.

Whether the patient dies at home or in the hospital, this is the end of the patient career. Although autopsies may be done or body parts removed for transplant, the patient is obviously no longer involved in decision-making.

CHAPTER 5

THE PATIENT AS A VICTIM

In his book *Victimology*, Schafer (1968) developed a system of categorization for victims of crimes and provided examples of each category of victim. He was trying to demonstrate that crimes and criminals cannot be understood in the absence of an understanding of the victim.

A victim is defined as the recipient of an injurious act or event. Victims of crimes may also be victimized by the judicial system itself. Women, for example, continue to be victimized by the courts in cases of rape. Whether the rapist is given an extremely reduced sentence because he is a young athlete, a lawyer implies the victim did not try hard enough to protect herself by demonstrating how difficult it is to thread a moving needle, or the judge tells the victim she needed to keep her knees crossed, the women in these examples are being doubly victimized by both the criminal and the justice system.

Patients, too, can be defined as the receivers of some form of injury (i.e., victims), whether from a pathogen/disease, an accident, a negative judgmental attitude, or a deliberate act. Just as individuals can be potential patients, actual patients, or former patients, they can also be potential, actual, or former victims. Being alive is risky. Everyone is a potential victim.

There are, however, different connotations to being a victim of a crime and the victim of a disease. Being the victim of a crime carries with it the suspicion that the victim might somehow have "brought it on himself." Being a patient does not carry that negative connotation. Very few Americans believe anyone would want to be a patient; being a patient is being helpless and defenseless in the face of possible disfigurement, disability, or death. Normally, patiency is to be avoided, if possible. Although people do become patients when seeking elective surgery, the goal is not patiency. Unsuccessful suicides frequently become patients, but again, the goal is not patiency.

Based on the typology presented in *Victimology*, the initial typology of patients as victims of their pathologies is presented below:

The Patient as a Victim of Pathology
The Innocent Victim: When the victim of a crime is totally innocent, the criminal is held fully responsible for the criminal act. If, however, a defense counsel can demonstrate the victim had some involvement in the crime, the criminal's responsibility is reduced. In criminology, the innocent victim is the individual who is believed to have no conscious or unconscious drives toward tempting the criminal act. Children and the mentally challenged are usually believed to be innocent. The adult who has taken steps to prevent accident or injury is also considered innocent. In any criminal trial, defense counsel makes every attempt to discredit the innocence of the victim.

The Patient as Innocent Victim: In health care, patients are believed to be "innocent" of having any involvement in causing their disease or injury until proven otherwise. With the advent of greater knowledge of disease causation, certain diseases once believed to have been patient caused have been redefined as innocent. Genetic anomalies, some viral or bacterial infections, and aging are all considered innocent conditions; patients with these and similar conditions are, therefore, considered innocent victims. And patients are always considered innocent victims when the health problem is caused by the health-care provider (iatrogenic diseases) or by the environment (exposure to asbestos, contaminated water supplies, or defective sewage systems). Children are always considered innocent patients.

The Simulating Victim: This is a person who claims to be the victim of a crime but for whom no criminal act can be found. Examples come from the fable "The Boy Who Cried Wolf." A person who wishes to claim enormous monetary recompense for an essentially minor or nonexistent accident and a paranoid schizophrenic who sees enemies everywhere are examples of simulating victims. A simulating victim can destroy lives when accusing others of a crime where none existed. Many women have unfairly been accused of being simulating victims in rape trials.

The Patient as a Simulating Victim: These are the people who "shop around" to find a physician who will treat their imaginary illnesses. This is especially true of people who have become addicted to their pain medications and have trouble finding a physician to renew their prescriptions. Some long-term patients are so comfortable in their role as patient that any threat of discharge will bring on a new set of symptoms. Rosenhahn conducted a study (Rosenhahn 1973) in which he created simulating victims to test the validity of psychiatric diagnoses. Rosenhahn invited volunteers for his study and gave them a list of symptoms to give the admitting physician. If they were admitted to a psychiatric ward, they were to behave normally (in other words, be their usual selves). Rosenhahn called his volunteers "Pseudo-patients." When they were admitted to an in-patient psychiatric ward, they were accepted by staff as "real patients." The volunteers did not display or complain of the symptoms they gave at their admitting interview. Staff never questioned the admitting diagnosis. In fact, a few of the volunteers needed Rosenhahn to explain the study to the staff so they could be discharged. Most of his volunteers were not discovered to be what he called "pseudo-patients." It is a fascinating study that created a firestorm of criticism. On follow-up, Rosenhahn found fewer people were being admitted using the symptoms he used in his study.

Another type of patient who might be categorized as a simulating victim is the person from a non-Western culture. People from other cultures have different ideas about the causes of illnesses and may come to a health agency with a list of confusing symptoms. The symptoms are meaningful to the patient but not to the provider. If the patient is an immigrant, that person will have different expectations of the healer, the facility, and the treatment plan. When the healer and patient do not share the same worldview of the causes and treatments of diseases, the patient is frequently classified as simulating a health issue.

The simulating patient is not as toxic as the simulating victim in criminology. Even when the physician suspects a patient is simulating, there is always doubt. There are illnesses that have not yet been diagnosed and symptomologies too obscure to diagnose. Until the simulating patient is proven beyond a shadow of a doubt to have manufactured the problem, that person should be retained within the health- care delivery system (HCDS). There are too many stories of people being labeled simulating Patient only to be found later that they had a valid pathogen that had not been discovered. The cause of pain, for example, can be obscure and difficult to trace.

The Careless Victim: In criminology, the careless victim is the person who goes away on holiday without leaving a light on or stopping the newspaper delivery. Careless victims do not think ahead to protect their property or themselves. Texting while driving is extreme carelessness with the possibility of causing injury or death to oneself and others.

The Patient as a Careless Victim: The careless patient in health care is the accident victim who did not fasten the seatbelt, did not clean up a spill on the floor, was not paying attention when using knives, and so on. Carelessness also applies to the care of medications, not reading labels, and not storing food or poisons properly. Today, the mobile game *Pokémon Go* has led to people walking in front of cars or over cliffs, causing injury or even death. Distracted driving leads to automobile accidents. Refusing to wear a helmet while operating a bicycle or motorcycle can lead to death or brain injuries.

The Provoker Victim: In criminology, the provoker victim is the individual who deliberately provokes a criminal attack. The person who challenges someone with an "I dare you" is inviting trouble. Bullies may find themselves attacked. Frequently, the provoker victim is considered more culpable than the criminal.

The Patient as a Provoker Victim: The provoker patient in health care is looked at with suspicion. Teasing or baiting dogs can lead to dog bites and even rabies. Drug abuse, alcoholism, obesity, and smoking are all classed as provoker behaviors. Someone who has unprotected sex with a known carrier of a sexually transmitted disease (STD) is a provoker. The provoker patient is playing Russian roulette with his or her future health. These patients are seen as deliberately contributing to their own disease causation. Provoker patients are seen as persisting in deviant or socially devalued behaviors if they overdose or develop lung cancer, an STD, or cirrhosis of the liver. At one time, staff refused to care for patients with AIDS as there was no known cure, and method of transmittal was obscure. These patients are frequently seen as not really deserving of care. The person who delays seeking treatment for ongoing symptoms may be considered as either a provoker or as careless.

These patients tend to persist in the behaviors that brought them to the clinic. Staff do not like or appreciate recidivism, repeated admissions for the same problem caused by the patient. Staff question whether the patients even deserve to be admitted or treated.

The Voluntary Victim: This is the individual who agrees to, or cooperates with, the criminal act. They are seen as being equally as guilty as the criminal. Before assisted suicide was judged to be legal, both physician and patient were considered criminals. Some people consider battered women to be voluntary victims as they do not leave the abusive situation readily.

The Patient as a Voluntary Victim: Voluntary victim patients includes those who voluntarily seek health care or elective surgeries. They also participate in physician-assisted suicide, suicide, and/or volunteer for medical experiments whether or not they have a disease.

The Potential Victim: In criminology, "victims at risk" refers to the fact that all individuals are potential victims of a crime. Certain variables increase the probability of becoming a victim. The differences in risk include time of day (nighttime is a higher risk), summer versus winter, and urban versus rural, among other considerations. The type of crime differs between strangers, family members, and business associates. The number of people involved also changes the character of the crime.

The Patient as a Potential Victim: As with the potential victim, the potential patient also includes everyone. Every human being is at potential risk of developing a disease or injury sometime in life. Certain populations are at higher risk than others. A person's age, gender, race, and environmental circumstances predispose him or her to certain diseases and injuries. Many carcinogens are linked to the environment, age, or gender. Communicable diseases can be predicted from a knowledge of age and environmental situation. The risk of automobile accidents is higher in some age groups than others. Many stress reactions are now predictable based on an analysis of life changes. Community health and preventive medicine services were created for potential patients.

Staff Value Judgments and Expectations Based upon Victim Category

Health professionals make value judgments about the quality and quantity of health care they will offer to patients based on an assessment of the degree of responsibility for the pathology. These value judgments are made on a sliding scale that dictates preferential treatment. In the hospital emergency room, patients are categorized by degree of trauma, time of admission, and victim status. A small boy playing with a gun shoots himself in the head. He will probably be taken care of more quickly than an old man who shoots himself in the head in an attempted suicide. Triage by victim status is an unconscious assessment.

A victim typology can provide a base for predicting patient-staff interactions as well as the degree to which the patient will be expected to participate in care. Staff respond most favorably to the innocent victim. Staff can also relate to careless victims, who are negligent, or ignorant. The provoker victim, however, would be relabeled as "self-induced" and, therefore, considered to be less deserving of time and attention. The simulating victim is viewed with ambivalence since some undiscovered pathogen might be causing the symptoms.

Expected patient behaviors are directly related to victim status. The innocent victim is expected to participate fully with treatment and desire a full cure. The careless person can also be negligent about eliminating hazards around the home that can cause accidents. Whether the person was ignorant of what caused the health problem, that person is expected to comply with treatment as well since the disease was not consciously desired. Simulating and provoker victims are viewed with suspicion. The rate of recidivism in these groups is high. Provokers may participate in care but are believed to be less than honest in their desire to be free of the pathology that caused the symptoms.

Since it is the HCDS that decides which patients will be accepted for services and since treatment is frequently predicated on the patient's status as victim, there is increasing need to clarify the position of the patient within the health system.

What is the point in having a victim typology in health care? Just as victims of crimes can also be victims of the judicial system, victims of pathology can also be victims of the system created to treat and heal them.

The Patient as a Victim of the Health-Care Delivery System

We are all familiar with the stories of surgeries in which surgical instruments were left in the patient's abdomen. These stories are rare, but they reflect the tunnel vision of practitioners. One woman had a noticeable growth on her face that kept growing. Although she asked her physician about it at every physical exam, she was told, "Just keep your hands away from it." One year, the MD tried liquid nitrogen on it with no appreciable result. It was her periodontist, who checked annually for lumps and bumps, who asked about this growth and what had been done about it. He asked if she would like a referral to a dermatologist, and she said she would. He gave her the referral, explaining that if the growth was benign, health insurance would not cover the removal. The growth turned out to be a squamous-cell carcinoma. The GP had simply ignored an obvious health issue that turned out to be cancerous. Why? He had tunnel vision. He was obviously focused on something else and glossed over a serious problem.

A chiropractor told the story of her daughter who had just had a baby. Her daughter complained to her OB/GYN about pain in her abdomen while she was pregnant. He dismissed the pain as "just the baby kicking." The pain continued. She had a cesarean section and delivered a healthy baby. When she complained to the nurses of the pain in her stomach, they said it was just the stitches. She was discharged, still in pain. When a nurse heard this story, she said, "Call your GP immediately!" The nurse told her to tell her GP that she had pain in her "right lower quadrant that would not go away and was getting worse."

She called the GP. Suspecting she had appendicitis, he made a referral to a surgeon. Her appendix, which had burst, was removed, and IV antibiotics were started. She could have died because her OB/GYN and the nursing staff on the maternity ward had tunnel vision. All they were interested in was her pregnancy, a normal delivery, and a healthy baby. When the chiropractor complained to the regional medical association, she was told that her daughter could not sue the MD for malpractice because she had not died.

In another situation, an elderly couple sought medical advice for potential Alzheimer's disease. Both were still active, living at home and caring for themselves; held valid driver's licenses; and drove daily. They wanted an assessment of some symptoms they had noticed that were relatively mild. After the man's exam, the physician said, "Don't go home. Go directly to the Alzheimer's facility and check yourself in." This abrupt and unfeeling statement was met with shock and confusion. The diagnosis sounded final and was devastating. The physician's attitude was much too callous and detached. Clearly the physician was not paying attention to the patient as a person; he did not make the connection between his assessment that the patient was so mentally challenged that he belonged in a secure inpatient facility and that the patient had driven himself to the appointment.

A fifty-year-old, grossly obese woman was admitted to a medical ward. During the night, she fell out of bed. The night staff scolded her, saying, "If we try to get you back in bed, we will injure our backs. You fell out; you get yourself back in." Eight hours later the woman died. She was still on the floor. The medical committee that reviews hospital deaths decided she had died of alcohol poisoning, despite there being no alcohol in her system.

These are examples of the patient being a victim of the health-care delivery system. They are also examples of staff attitudes, tunnel vision, and iatrogenic issues (Steiger 1964). When the provider fails to make a correct diagnosis because of tunnel vision, it clearly demonstrates the need for a more holistic approach to diagnosis and treatment. These examples also illustrate that the patient has no recourse when the physician does not act in his or her best interest.

The Patient as a Victim of Staff Attitudes

In addition to making value judgments, health professionals "like" some patients and not others. This puts health-care providers in a bind because they must act as if they like the people they don't. There is an unspoken rule that all patients are equal and have equal rights to competent and expert health care. Anyone who has worked in health care knows that the sicker the patient and the more critical, the higher the priority for care. Priority of needs trumps equality for care and attention.

As previously discussed, staff attitudes toward patients are colored by their beliefs about the degree to which the patient is responsible for the health problem. Negative attitudes of personnel toward patients can result in mutual avoidance, limited or ineffective health care, or even death, as the example of the obese woman demonstrates. Raising staff awareness of their own unconscious attitudes toward patients, based on victimology, might improve health-care services (Steiger 1964).

Patients' Families as Victims of Staff Attitudes

An old woman lived in an inpatient, long-term-care facility. She had been bedridden for so long that she had developed contractures of both legs and could not stand or walk. She was admitted to an acute-care hospital for eye surgery. When visited by her daughter after her surgery, a young man came into her room and began to give her evening nursing care. The daughter introduced herself, assuming he was her primary nurse, and started to tell him about her mother's contractures and deafness, in case he had been newly assigned to her care.

He whipped around and looked directly at the daughter, saying, "I am so tired of you being so superior and telling me what to do. No one can stand you on this ward because you are so demanding." This was the first time she had seen this young man. She was shocked. Somehow, she had gotten a label by the nursing staff as an interfering relative. The young man was obviously angry at her even though they had never met. She never did find out how she got the label of being a difficult and interfering family member. Talking to the director of nursing had little effect. Thankfully, her mother was discharged the next day.

Families can be victims of staff attitudes about patient privacy. Family members may be excluded from knowing what the healer and patient discussed. Friends are even more likely to be ignored. In one instance, a physician shooed out three friends who were visiting. The physician planned to examine the patient and discuss the findings with her. When the three friends came back in the room, they asked, "What did he say? Did he tell you what was wrong with you? Can you come home tomorrow?"

The patient slowly shook her head, saying, "I am still trying to absorb it all. I can't remember everything he said."

From the next bed, a voice popped up and said, "Why don't you ask me? I heard the whole thing." Four heads turned in unison to the lady in the next bed. A total stranger. The physician had asked friends and family to leave while he talked to his patient but had not bothered to lower his voice. He dismissed the patient in the next bed as irrelevant.

Patients sharing a room cannot help but overhear conversations. Boredom and lack of diversion prompt them to listen, but out of politeness, they do not acknowledge they are listening intently.

So two strangers become intimately involved while three friends, anxious to know what is going on, are left in ignorance.

Patients as Victims of Iatrogenic Pathology
A psychologist once said at a convention that "eighty percent of the diseases currently being treated in hospitals are iatrogenic diseases." "Iatrogenic" means the disease was caused by the health-care system. He went on to say, "Iatrogenic diseases are the number-one health problem in the United States. There are more iatrogenic diseases than the other leading diseases: cancer, heart disease, and obesity."

If, in fact, iatrogenic diseases are the leading health problem in the United States, then patients are indeed victims—victims of a health-care delivery system designed for the care and cure of diseases.

How is it that a system designed to cure and control disease causes disease? Very simply. Health professionals are human beings who make mistakes. Even with highly sophisticated technology, mistakes are made.

Thalidomide babies are a case in point. A drug designed to relieve one symptom, morning sickness, produced an unintended and unanticipated consequence: birth defects. Thalidomide babies were victims of the system.

With the increase in medical technology has come an increase in iatrogenic diseases. At one time, premature babies were automatically placed in incubators and given 100 percent oxygen. Later it was discovered that these babies developed blindness.

Premature babies who have been kept alive have been found to have genetic anomalies that might have triggered the spontaneous abortion. Individuals suffering severe brain damage from accidents or drug overdoses are now being kept alive. This ability to maintain life in an essentially brain dead individual, raises many issues, not just for the family but for the HCDS as well. There are the questions about, "When is a person dead? What are the criteria? Who decides? Is survival on life support, keeping an essentially dead person alive? If, on the remote chance that the person does wake up, how do they live with their brain injury? Where will they be cared for? Who pays for the care? Medical technology has improved many lives and raised questions about others. People have developed entirely new diseases as side effects of medical experiments. This was especially true prior to medical ethics review boards for medical research.

Physicians and health-care facilities are now being sued for medical procedures that had unintended consequences. Many law firms specialize in suing the medical profession. Even though the patient is buying into the current medical knowledge and expertise, treatment is always risky. The patient and the physician enter a contract for services based on all the facts available at the time. New facts and treatments come out daily. What is known today can be replaced, disproved, or enhanced tomorrow. The patient can expect the physician to diagnose and treat based only on what is currently known, not on what might become known. Nevertheless, the patient trusts that the physician is up to date on current treatment choices. Ignorance of current medical knowledge is a failure of both physicians and the HCDS.

The patient who becomes a victim of an iatrogenic disease caused by current (but insufficient) medical knowledge is indeed a victim but an unintended victim. Physicians, however, are not the only ones who cause iatrogenic diseases.

One of the administrators of a Nigerian medical school once told me the school had received notice from the state government that all enrolled medical students were to graduate and receive their medical degrees regardless of their performance. No one was to be failed. This government interference in medical education happened because there was a paucity of physicians. This short-sighted government decree, intended to deal with one problem, meant the citizens had a lower quality of medical care. Medical mistakes that resulted from this decision must be laid at the door of the government, not the medical profession.

At one time, schools of nursing were attached to hospitals. The purpose of the school was to produce well-trained personnel for the hospital. After a six-month probationary period in which the student was taught about diseases and their treatments, they were placed on ward duty for the rest of their three years. There they received practical experience on all shifts and on all wards. Students were closely supervised and dismissed for mistakes. The hospital only wanted the best graduates.

Today in the United States, nursing is taught in college and university programs. Course work is integrated with clinical practice. Few, if any, students are failed or dismissed for mistakes or poor-quality work. Nursing faculty tend to feel sorry for the student who does not do well and do everything in their power to help the poor student succeed. The consequence is providing poorer-quality nurses to the community. With the growing complexity of the HCDS, mistakes can be made by anyone employed by the system. Health-care delivery systems employ many kinds of health-care professionals and paraprofessionals, as well as ancillary workers who keep the facility running. Each group educates, qualifies, and monitors its own graduates. The facility hires these graduates assuming they are qualified to do the work. Yet the quality of the training and experience of these employees is variable. The facility loosely monitors its employees for quality of care.

Mistakes are made by all groups at one time or another. A mistake can be made in blood typing for surgery. The wrong kidney can be removed. Scissors can be left in an abdomen during surgery. Hallways can be slippery. Catheters and other supplies can be contaminated. Staff may not sufficiently wash their hands or their patient's wounds. The variety of possible mistakes is enormous. The patient, the receiver of the facility's services, is under the total control of the facility from admission to discharge. Any human being under the total control of other human beings is in danger of being victimized in one way or another.

Since the 1970s, when this book was originally written, there has been a shift in the thinking about what constitutes a healthy diet. "The Dietary Guidelines for Americans" (which comes out every five years) was rewritten in 1980 to reflect the dietary hypothesis at the time. Based largely on untested findings, Americans have been advised to eat less meat, particularly red meat, and less saturated fat (usually associated with meats) and eat more fruits, vegetables, and grains. This dietary advice was based on a concern for preventing heart disease. Since those recommendations came out, however, there has been an appalling increase not only in heart disease but also in diabetes, high blood pressure, cancer, and obesity. Although subsequent research has refuted these guidelines' effectiveness, the same dietary recommendations have been repeated in every report. And Americans have been doing a good job following these them. (An outstanding literature review on the medical research and politics involved in producing these dietary guidelines was written by Gary Taubes (2007).

"The Dietary Guidelines for Americans" of 2010 and 2015 have not changed significantly since the publication of Taubes' book.

This dietary solution, based on inadequate medical research and knowledge, appears to have created the problems it was designed to control. The sad fact is, the medical establishment refuses to look at these results and do any research to prove or disprove their hypothesis (Teicholtz 2015). Instead, the medical literature continues to reaffirm its position that a diet high in carbohydrates (fruits, grains, and vegetables) and low in protein and fats (especially animal fats) is the diet most Americans should eat. Despite taking the Hippocratic oath to "do no harm" and undergoing scientific training to examine every discrepant finding, the medical community has done little to systematically study this issue. Once again, the question arises: Whose needs are being served?

Patients as Victims of Neglect
A young woman was injured in an automobile accident and taken to the nearest emergency room. She was in a state of shock and could not remember what medical insurance she had. She lay on a stretcher for two hours without treatment, until she finally remembered the telephone number of her boyfriend. When called, he immediately came and took her to another hospital. Only when she remembered her medical insurance was she admitted for treatment at that hospital. Although she had obvious cuts and bruises and an X-ray revealed broken bones, she was not considered a patient until she could guarantee payment for services. Her pain was ignored.

In another hospital, a young woman was brought by ambulance after an attempted suicide by drug overdose. "You'll just have to wait," the emergency-room nurse told her. "There are other patients who really need us!" The young woman remained unattended for hours.

Patients as Victims of Socially Devalued Pathology
People who have come to the emergency room as attempted suicides have told me they were treated with negligence, if not complete avoidance. This treatment is not limited to suicidal patients. Alcoholics, drug addicts, the obese, gays, and transgendered people have told me they have experienced this level of avoidance as well. What they have in common is that their issues are all considered socially deviant behaviors or the results of them. Social values are frequently carried over to health-care situations. If another patient is "sicker," then that patient will receive the attention, and

the other patients must wait. Patients are expected to understand and accept this as well.

One socially devalued health problem is obesity. Obese people are commanded to lose weight prior to surgery with no apparent understanding or appreciation for their history with weight control. Telling them to lose weight prior to surgery and expecting compliance borders on psychotic thinking. There is a disconnect between the reality of the patient's inability to lose weight and the health-care personnel's desire that the patient follow orders. The obese badly need Patientologists. Someone who has had weight-control issues has more understanding and sympathy for all the problems surrounding obesity and weight loss. Those who have not had this experience think obesity is controlled by simply not eating so much! The simplistic attitude toward the obese is like the attitudes toward alcoholics and addicts.

Patients as Victims of Their Social Status
Patients may be "bumped" from their place in line by a person of higher social status. A politician, famous athlete, or movie star will be treated before anyone else. Patients are expected to understand and accept that some patients are more important than others. Not only are patients expected to be understanding, but they are expected to be docile. Unfortunately, these are not unusual situations.

Negative attitudes of health-care professionals toward their patients can result in mutual avoidance, limited or ineffective health care, or death. The need to change negative attitudes in health care has ramifications for the health system as well as for all major social systems that directly or indirectly interact with the health system. Health professionals must be constantly alert to their own negative attitudes and their subsequent behavior because of these attitudes.

If there were a specialty area of Patientology in the health sciences, just as there is an area of victimology in criminology, one major avenue of research could be "The Patient as Victim." This area of research would include 1) the patient as victim of their pathology and 2) the patient as a victim of the health-care delivery system.

To review, the patient as a victim of the HCDS includes the study of staff attitudes based on victim typology, socially devalued pathologies, and iatrogenic (caused by the HCDS) problems. The study of the patient as a victim of pathology can also be viewed based on the victim typology.

Other Victim Types
It's not possible to present in detail all possible victim types, but a few others are worth a brief mention. There are acquisitive, biological, depressed, guilty, heartbroken, imprudent, lonesome, passive, tormentor, and wanton victims. Some neatly dovetail into the victim types previously described. Others require more research. Each descriptive category does have some value for further analysis of the patient as a victim. These victim types have been based on the work of Schafer (1968), who was working on other victim typologies that might interest health-care workers, such as the victim subculture. Just as new concepts regarding the relationship between the victim and the criminal contribute to the field of victimology, the role of patient-as-victim might produce new insights into a field of Patientology.

The Typology of Patient-as-Victim Raises Additional Questions
The concept of patient-as-victim is not satisfied by a simple typology. Rather, this concept leads to a different set of questions about staff-patient interactions that could be explored. Although there are many studies of staff attitudes toward patients in different pathological categories, would these attitude studies be enhanced

by an examination of a staff's own categorization of these patients as victims? Do staff know they are judging patients by one or the other of these victim types? Because the quality of health care appears to be determined by victim types, are there other factors that influence the quality of care? Do patients' demographic characteristics also influence their classification as victims? As we have seen, age and gender influence placement in the system, but will ethnic origin, immigrant status, or language facility also influence victim typology? Only research can answer these questions.

Of what use is a victim typology for patients? Is there a difference in behavior patterns between one type of victim and another? Is there more compliance from the innocent victim than the simulating victim? Or vice versa?

Do patients perceive themselves as victims? If so, how would they define their own victim status? If all patients believe themselves to be innocent victims, on what basis would they judge or explain neglect, rudeness, or personalized attention? On what basis do patients select their physicians, rate nursing care, or miss outpatient appointments? Can any of these questions be answered using the patient-as-victim concept?

Another approach might be to view the patient-as-victim from a positive or negative valuation of victim types. Which victim types are the most positively valued, which are negatively valued, and which have ambivalent connotations? Would it make a difference if the patient or the health-care provider were doing the evaluating? Which victim types would be considered legitimate? Is there a strong correlation between the patient's responsibility for disease causation and cooperation with treatment?

These questions, as well as many others, were stimulated by the concept of patient-as-victim. The concept does seem to have a bearing on the rights and privileges of patients in health-care settings. Research should be done to support or disprove the idea or to determine whether the concept has any practicality at all.

CHAPTER 6
THE PATIENT'S PERSPECTIVE

Everyone has a slightly different idea of what health care is all about. Whether patients, health professionals, recent immigrants, or Mayflower descendants, they all hold firmly held beliefs about what health care is, what it should be, and how it can be changed. Everyone is an expert. Can they all be right?

The Patient's View from outside the System
The American public has been taught to believe that health care is the right of all citizens, is uniformly available, and is delivered at the highest level of professional competence to all who request it. For most people, the hospital is where they go when they are very sick or in need of surgery. They also have many idealized beliefs about the hospital: The hospital contains the most modern technology that can cure almost any ailment as well as physicians who are personally and deeply committed to their profession; who are nationally recognized as the best in their fields; and who are clean, morally upright, respectful, and kind. To assist the physicians, there are beautiful nurses who wear white uniforms and look like angels. It is the nurse who holds the patient's hand, gently wipes off the perspiration, and cries when the patient dies heroically.

Then there is the laboratory technician who is capable of drawing blood efficiently, starting an IV, taking a chest X-ray, and administering CPR. The hospital is the stuff of fairy tales.

The patient's perspective is a direct result of his or her placement within the health-care system. The patient is an outsider, not a member of the team. Since the patient is receiving service, the type of service and the way the service is delivered will color the patient's perspective of the HCDS. Children, for example, are often fearful and can react with tears and stubbornness in the face of quick, efficient care. Gentleness produces a different result. Similarly, adults do not respond well to abrupt commands without explanation. Adults respond better if they are talked to nicely, if time is taken to explain and answer their questions, and if interest is shown to them personally. They appreciate explanations in answer to questions, a show of interest, and kindness. Patients do not expect a show of irritability or harsh treatment.

There are several published qualitative research studies and personal narratives on the patient's experience with the HCDS. These studies demonstrate the place of the patient as an outsider, as a necessary but inconvenient part of work. The usual criticism of these studies is their lack of generalizability. They are often ignored as just one person's experience.

What Shapes the Patient's View from the Outside?
The perspective of the potential patient (the outsider) is derived from personal experiences, school, books, magazines, television programs and ads, cultural background, movies, newspapers, and the Internet. Each media has a different reporting style, a different target audience, and different requirements for selling its product. The emphasis on the style of reporting health care, as well as the content, will differ with the type of media.

Novels and plays always have a dramatic plotline, at least one crises, a hero or heroine the reader can relate to, and a climactic scene in which all crises and plotlines are brought to a head and successfully resolved. For these stories, it is the drama that grips attention. Characters seem real. Here we find the superhuman physician who acts as both healer and nurse, is equally conversant with psychiatry and orthopedic surgery, invents a cure for the disease, performs cardiac transplants, and creates a new hospital department—all in the same episode. No one dies, but if they do die, it is after the doctor's heroic efforts to keep them alive. The minor characters all support the main character, the physician, with equal selflessness. Everyone is kind, considerate, likeable, and deferential.

This is the art of the novelist and script writers: making the fiction seem like reality. The public, with no real experience, will have their perspective of the HCDS colored by these stories.

The news media, on the other hand, presents a different picture. Although there are periodic stories of heroic hospital staff, the majority of stories are negative. Negativity and shock value sell. Stories about mistakes or immorality make the front page along with breakthroughs. Potential patients are influenced by stories of mistaken diagnoses, long wait times in emergency rooms, fake doctors, and other dramatic mishaps.

This essentially negative view of the HCDS is as distorted as the positive fictional stories. They highlight only one area of the system and ignore the daily humdrum of everyday care. But potential patients will make decisions about seeking care based on this information.

The TV documentary or the nonfiction expose book blend the fictional requirement of an interesting plotline with the reality of the situation. Even documentaries and books have a slant they are selling. The drama is still paramount.

The potential patient is confronted by a plethora of confusing messages about the HCDS and health professionals. Who do they trust? Who do they believe?

This, then, is the dilemma as well as the view of the potential patient from outside the system. Without prior experience, a potential patient may have a completely distorted point of view. Potential patients' expectations are colored by what they have heard, read, or seen on TV. For some, these perceptions prevent them from knowingly seeking health care, regardless of their symptomology. For others, long-lasting pain is the only thing that will make them seek care. Religious beliefs prevent others from seeking care, even when they have a communicable disease or are facing impending death. For the inexperienced potential patient, the fear and uncertainty surrounding the diagnosis and treatment of physical symptoms might make them delay too long in seeking help.

The Patient's View from the Bottom
In the organizational chart of health-care delivery services, the patient is either assumed to exist and does not appear on the chart or is placed at the bottom of the chart as the recipient of services.

In total-care, long-term facilities, the patient's perspective is largely ignored (Goffman 1961). Staff have been known to bully patients or deliberately neglect them. Negatively valued patients or those stigmatized by having a health problem believed to be self-induced are at the greatest risk for mistreatment (see chapter 4). Staff have been known to steal patient drugs but chart that the drugs have been administered. When patients complain that they have not received their medications or that their pain medication was not effective, it is the chart—not the patient—that is believed.

In many ways, admission to a hospital is very much like culture shock (Brink 1990). The hospital culture is very different from either the culture of the home or the wider community. Communication systems use utterly foreign words and phrases, customary forms of behavior are interrupted, beliefs and values are foreign, there is isolation from families and friends, and totally different forms of technology are present.

The staff hierarchy can be confusing; patients tend to lump hospital personnel into broad categories. Any man wearing surgical greens or a white uniform with a stethoscope draped around his neck is perceived as a doctor whether he is or not. Women in surgical greens or white uniforms with stethoscopes draped around their necks are all believed to be nurses whether they are or not. Despite the influx of women into medicine and men into nursing since the '70s, most patients see women as nurses and men as doctors.

All employees of a health-care facility, from admitting clerks to housekeeping staff, are considered "the hospital." Any negative treatment of the patient will be the hospital's fault.

Patients are quite willing to express their opinions about their care. In published interviews with patients or their families, several stated they did not agree with the treatment prescribed by the physician. When asked to describe what they believed to be the bad nursing care they received, they said, "I had to wait around for the nurses," or, "The nurses seemed unconcerned and gave no explanations." Nurses were described as being bossy, acting like policemen, scolding, being rude, and treating the patient like a child. Some nurses were criticized for giving the wrong medicine or the wrong dose. Still others complained that when two nurses were giving care, they talked to each other rather than the patient. In yet another example, a bedridden patient was given a bedpan, but after half an hour of waiting for someone to remove it, she tried getting rid of it herself, resulting in spillage.

What Shapes the Patient's View from the Bottom?
The patient's view of health care is affected by pain, fear, horror stories, experience, and uncertainty. Not knowing what to expect colors everything. Feeling ill changes perspectives and attention spans, blocking out all instructions and information.

When patients feel ill or in pain, their ability to focus on anything else is limited. They have trouble concentrating on what they are being told and can't remember explanations or instructions. They are faced with a terrible uncertainty: Will they live or die? If they live, will they be permanently disabled, or will it be temporary? Fear of the unknown or of what to expect colors everything. Thus, patients can become demanding, uncooperative, or irritable.

The patient's perspective will be colored by many factors not even touched on here. For example, the patient's religious beliefs can have an enormous impact or none. The patient's culture (French 1973) and profession will also color his or her expectations for care.

Julius Roth, a medical sociologist, spent a year in a tuberculosis sanatorium. His description of the experience is informative. He was generally critical of the nursing care he received (Roth 1963).

In contrast, good nursing care was described as the staff checking on the patients frequently; giving competent and efficient care; taking time to answer questions; and being kind, helpful, concerned, and available. Good staff are those who are attentive to patient needs. A good nurse will understand that when a patient must lie flat on his or her back all day and all night, a backrub would be appreciated. A poor nurse does not even notice.

Most patients are content with the care and treatment they receive. A few are angry or resentful toward hospital personnel—especially physicians and nurses. Whether the patients' perception of the care they receive is distorted by pain, ignorance, fear, or medications, the distorted view exists and must be attended to immediately. It cannot wait.

The Insider's View from the Inside
The health professional who becomes a patient has a different set of expectations from other patients. The health professional, whether a dentist, nurse, or physician, knows the types of mistakes

that can be made, knows what happens on the other side of the door, and understands the color coding and PA system codes. They know the degree to which staff can be pushed or pulled. They know because they have been there.

There is a great deal of difference between advising patients to change their unhealthy habits and doing it yourself. There is a difference between doing a procedure and having it done to you. The health professional may know more but will be just as uninterested in being a patient as anyone else and is likely to be even more critical and demanding.

Compared with others, health professionals are more likely to follow health prescriptions such as exercising, watching their diet, and not smoking. Thus, they are touchier when other health professionals do not respect their judgment or qualifications.

The Family's Perspective
Standing between the patient and health-care personnel are family, friends, and lovers who can be fearful, uncomfortable, helpless, defensive, and angry. They are the buffer between the patient and the system. They are protectors. The family believes that they, and they alone, stand guard over the patient—that it is they who are most concerned over the patient's rights and welfare. It is they who are personally involved, personally concerned. (Richardson 1945),

The patient's significant others have a decidedly different view of the system from either the patient or the caregivers. Depending on their emotional attachment to the patient, their reactions will differ. Spouses have been known to have helpless rage reactions: screaming or shouting, berating the physician for letting their wife or husband die. Some, reacting to their fears, abandon their relative to the hospital and caregivers. Gay couples have been at a distinct disadvantage when their partners are in the ICU because only "family members" are allowed to visit.

Significant others, including spouses, parents, and children, among others, are in a tenuous position. They have no place in the system; they are outsiders. They have no role, no status, no say. Because of this uncertainty of position, family are asked to leave the room when basic care is being given or when the physician wishes to examine the patient. Family may want to help but have no idea whether what they do will help or hurt.

A grossly obese woman was diagnosed with cancer of the esophagus, a fast-growing cancer. Although she was admitted to the local cancer center, her primary oncologist did not make an appointment to see her for four months. A friend of hers went to the hospital administrator, who happened to be a friend, and complained about this apparent neglect. An appointment was made with her primary oncologist the following week. At this visit, the patient and her family were informed that she needed a very specialized surgery that could not be performed at the local facility. She would need to travel thousands of miles to a different cancer facility. She and two of her sisters made the trip together. She survived the surgery, and one month after arrival, all three returned home. She lived less than a year following her surgery.

Why was there a delay in her treatment? Why did her oncologist neglect her? Was it because she was grossly obese or because the physician felt helpless about a condition he could not treat or cure? Did she die because of the neglect?

Families are usually helpless in the face of these situations. They have no clout, no recourse. Had this woman not had a friend who knew the administrator, she might have died much sooner and in great pain.

It is the health-care provider who is responsible for noting when there is a conflict in perceptions about care and when the patient's perspective might interfere with the treatment plan. The patient's perspective will influence progress through the HCDS. If the system takes notice and acts with understanding, the patient will be more cooperative, the experience will be more positive for both parties, and the outcome will hopefully be a success.

CHAPTER 7

A FINAL NOTE: TOWARD A SCIENCE OF PATIENTOLOGY

Patientology focuses on the human recipient of health care rather than the techniques, technologies, products, services, organizations, facilities, and efficiency of the health-care delivery system. It is not the education and experience of the provider that is the focus but the education and experience of the recipient—the patient. Rather than focusing on the diagnosis and treatment of pathology, Patientology focuses on the person who has the pathology and how he or she lives with it.

Patientology could provide a greater awareness of giver-receiver relationships and whether this form of contract, which occurs in business, also occurs in health care. In fact, there is an entire book that describes the patient as a "consumer" of health-care delivery services in much the same way as customers are described in businesses (Krizay 1974). In any relationship, both parties are important to study.

Patientology suggests an intimacy between provider and patient. It suggests the provider has a sense of what the patient is going through and respects the patient's feelings as valid. It suggests the provider understands what it is like to live with this pathology and its treatment. It suggests the patient is not an object to be acted on but a coparticipant in the healing process.

Since Patientology involves provider-patient interactions, a major research method for studying these interactions should be participant observation. Interviewing the provider reveals only what a provider thinks is happening. It is an idealized self-evaluation. Observation of the provider (perhaps filming the interaction) documents what really happens. In fact, filming an inpatient ward all day long would offer a great deal of information about the life of an inpatient, which would reveal the actions and interactions of the providers. Then the researcher can ask why certain things were done in a certain way.

In the same manner, interviewing patients about their inpatient hospital experiences will be colored by their perceptions of what is going on, how long they have been hospitalized, and what is wrong with them. The patients' evaluations will likely focus on the interpersonal relationships and the food rather than the quality of the technology.

What do patients think about when waiting in a waiting room for lab tests, diagnostic screening, prescriptions to be filled, or to be seen in the ER? What do they think about all day in a hospital bed? What do they think about as they are being discharged and going home? What do they think about when they have been home for one week posthospitalization? How do they evaluate their experiences at all stages of their health-care service? Does their pathology make a difference in their assessment? What of the duration of their hospital stay? Are there different perspectives based on age and gender? Could one person be followed from the discovery of symptoms, through diagnosis and treatment plan, hospitalization and discharge home? Are these studies even important?

Participant observation, while being more humanistic than interviewing, is generally considered "soft science," as the findings aren't mathematical. But it is participant observation that provides more information on what is happening than interviewing alone. The science of cultural anthropology is based on participant observation studies in which the researcher lives with the research subjects for a long period. The resulting publications give the reader a clear sense of who the people being observed are and what they are like. Research reports of a lifestyle are holistic. Anthropologists do not live in an apartment and drive to the field site. They live in a village with a family, sharing the food, games, courtesies, and duties of a family member. For example, Dr. Jean Hendry, an anthropologist, studied pottery-making in southern Mexico by living with a noted potter in his home. She felt she had "arrived" when she could take a bath with the other village women in the local river while the men wandered by and stared at this unusual white woman. Another anthropologist, Jill Salmons, lived in the home of a noted Annang carver in Nigeria, where she was able to observe him in his daily round of activity. Not only did she observe him in a family setting, but she saw when and where he worked, how he went about selling his products, who came to the compound to buy, and when he took his carvings to market. These intimate views of family life in a village setting provide a richer story than interviewing alone could have provided. Yet few researchers attempt this kind of study, seeing it as too time consuming.

Another area of research is self-monitoring. Health-care providers need to decide whether the service they provide is for self-gratification or for meeting patient needs. Being filmed all day long while interacting with patients would reveal what happens from day to day and would be a useful tool for self-critique. Providers could also keep a daily journal to be examined for trends and habitual practices. Granted, a daily journal is not as objective as a film, but it is one method of self-evaluation.

For some health providers, career advancement is their primary goal. The way they interact with patients is a secondary consideration to publications or administrative progression. In this case, colleagues might provide feedback. No one, however, enjoys criticism, so studies on this subject are unlikely to take place.

One way of including patients in health care is to invite them to serve on all health committees. For example, patients could be members of research teams. In an obesity-treatment research project, an obese or formerly obese person could be a member of the team to provide the patient's perspective. If the research is in the form of a questionnaire, the patient could provide patient-centered and patient-friendly questions. If the research is on bariatric surgery, a patient could provide questions about pre- and postsurgical experiences. If it is a clinical trial comparing different diet programs, a patient who has tried them all could provide insights that a researcher who has never been obese or on a diet might miss. What patients see as important in the care and treatment of their health problems may be ignored by a clinical researcher who has never experienced the problems firsthand.

Many clinicians see no value in any kind of research other than the clinical trial. What they don't realize is that there were many observational studies that preceded the clinical trial. Without observational studies, there would be no database necessary to design a clinical trial. These clinicians will probably balk at any suggestion for Patientology research protocols, much less having a patient on the research team. These are the clinicians who see patients as objects to be acted on and see the patients' perspectives as irrelevant. It's doubtful they would read Patientology research.

Perhaps research protocols could be designed to evaluate the patient-as-victim typology to see if this categorization is a valid observation. One such study could be a simple multiple-choice questionnaire. The situation could be an ER where the admitting nurse is asked to triage five patients who come in at the same time with identical injuries from accidents. They cannot all be seen at once. How does the nurse rank the patients to be seen first, second, and so on? Each patient can be given some of the characteristics listed in the patient-as-victim typology, according to the degree to which the patient caused his or her own accident. Then the nurse can be given the patients' demographic characteristics. The decision as to which patients should be seen first or last could provide a good discussion on how our attitudes affect our decisions. Such a study would reveal unspoken attitudes.

The concept of Patientology does not replace the current focus of health professionals, which is treating diseases. But it does add the patient dimension: a key element. Patientology is broadening. It is the health professional with a Patientology emphasis whom everyone respects and admires and returns to repeatedly. As any patient can attest, "You can have all the science in the world at your fingertips, but if you don't have heart, you don't have me as a patient."

REFERENCES

Abramson, Harold Alexander. 1956. *Mother Story Verbatim in Psychoanalysis of Allergic Illness.* New York: Vantage Press.
Bates, Richard C. 1968. *The Fine Art of Understanding Patients.* Ordale, NJ: Medical Economics. Book Division, Inc.
Brink, P. J. & Judith M. Saunders. 1990. "Culture Shock: Theoretical and Applied." In *Transcultural Nursing: A Book of Readings*, by P. J. Brink, 126–138. Reprinted by Waveland Press.
Brink, Pamela J. 1972. "Natural Triad in Health Care." *American Journal of Nursing* 72 (5): 897–899.
Brink, Pamela J. 1978. "Patientology: Just Another Ology?" *Nursing Outlook* 26 (9): 574–575.
Brink, Pamela. 1984. "The Patient as Victim." *American Journal of Nursing* 84 (7): 984.
Brink, Pamela J. 1985. "Editorial: On the Patient Role." *Western Journal of Nursing Research* 7 (4): 397–399.
Brink, Pamela J. 1991a. "Patientology One More Time." *Western Journal of Nursing Research* 13 (1): 9–11.
Brink, Pamela. 1991b. "When Patientology Is Ignored: The Case of Nazi Germany." *Western Journal of Nursing Research* 13 (2): 162–163.

Burgess, Ann Wolbert and Aaron Lazare. 1976. *Community Mental Health: Target Populations.* Englewood Cliffs, NJ: Prentice-Hall, Inc.

Cartwright, Ann. 1967. *Patients and Their Doctors.* London: Routledge and Keegan Paul.

Chapman, Jane E. & Harry H. Chapman. 1975. *Behaviors and Health Care: A Humanistic Helping Process.* Saint Louis: C. V. Mosby Co.

Chirco, Inice. 1963. *The Patient-Centered Approach to Nursing. Nurse Patient Relations.* New York: Brewster.

Field, Mark G. 1973. "The Concept of the 'Health System' at the Macrosociological Level." *Social Science and Medicine* 7: 763–785.

Field, Minnie. 1967. *Patients Are People: A Medical-Social Approach to Prolonged Illness.* New York: Columbia University Press.

Freilich, Morris. 1964. "The Natural Triad in Kinship and Complex Systems." *American Sociological Review* 29 (4): 529–540.

French, Jean & Schwartz, Doris R. 1973. "Terminal Care at Home in Two Cultures." *American Journal of Nursing* 73 (3): 502–5.

Goffman, Erving. 1961. *Asylums: Essays on the Social Situation of Mental Patients and Other Inmates.* Harpswell, ME: Anchor Books.

Greenblatt, M., D. J. Levinson, & R. Williams. 1957. *The Patient and the Mental Hospital.* Glencoe, IL: The Free Press.

Hochbaum, G. M. 1969. "Consumer Participation in Health Planning: Toward Conceptual Clarification." *American Journal of Public Health* 59 (9): 698–1705.

Hoffman, Lois. 1958. "Problem Patient: The Christian Scientist." In *Patients, Physicians and Illness*, edited by E. G. Jaco, 278–283. Glencoe, IL: The Free Press.

Hopkins, Phillip (ed.). 1972. *Patient-Centred Medicine.* London: Balint Society: Regional Dr Publications

Hoyle, Leigh. 1980. The Patient: Biological, Psychological, and Social Dimensions of Medical Practice. New York: Springer.

Hoyle, Leigh. 1981. "Patientology Exists-Reply." *Archives of Internal Medicine* 141 (8).

Jones, Ellen W. 1973. *Patient Classification for Long-Term Care.* Durham: McKnight.

Katz, D. & Kahn, R. L. 1964. "The Taking of Organizational Roles." *Social Psychology and Organizations* 171–198.

Krizay, John & Andrew Wilson. 1974. *The Patient as Consumer: Health Care Financing in the US.* Lexington: Lexington Books.

Ludvigsen, M. 2009. "Patient Life in Hospital: A Qualitative Study of Informal Relationships between Hospitalized Patients." PhD dissertation, The Department of Medicine and Nephrology C, Faculty of Health Sciences, Aarhus University.

Mayerson, Evelyn Wilde. 1976. *Putting the Ill at Ease.* New York: Harper & Row Publisher.

McGovern, John P. & Burns, Chester, R. Eds. 1973. *Humanism in Medicine.* Springfield: Charles C. Thomas, Publishers.

McGregor, Frances C. 1967. "Uncooperative Patients: Some Cultural Interpretations." *The American Journal of Nursing* 67 (1): 88–91.

Ramsey, Paul. 1970. *The Patient as a Person: Explorations in Medical Ethics.* New Haven, CT: Yale University Press.

Richardson, Henry B. 1945. *Patients Have Families.* New York: The Commonwealth Fund.

Robinson, George Canby. 1939. *The Patient as a Person: A Study of the Social Aspects of Illness.* New York: The Commonwealth Fund.

Rosenhahn, D. L. 1973. "On Being Sane in Insane Places." *Science* 179 (407): 250–58.

Roth, Juliu. 1963. *Timetables: Structuring the Passage of Time in Hospital Treatment and Other Careers.* New York: Bobbs-Merril.

Schafer, Stephen. 1968. *The Victim and His Criminal: A Study in Functional Responsibility.* New York: Random House, Inc.

Steiger, Willis. 1964. "Negative Attitudes of Health Care Professionals toward Their Patients Can Result in Mutual Avoidance." In *Patients Who Trouble You.*, by M. Anthony & Victor Hansen Jr. Boston: Little Brown.

Taubes, Gary. 2007. *Good Calories, Bad Calories.* New York: Knopf.
Teicholtz, Nina. 2014. *The Big Fat Surprise: Why Butter, Meat, and Cheese Belong in a Healthy Diet.* New York: Simon & Schuster.

ABOUT THE AUTHOR

Pamela J. Brink, RN, PhD, FAAN, was an associate professor of nursing and anthropology at UCLA, professor of nursing at the University of Iowa, and professor of nursing and anthropology at the University of Alberta. She has published many books and articles in the areas of nursing and anthropology. She initiated the *Western Journal of Nursing Research* and served as its editor for over twenty-five years.

www.ingramcontent.com/pod-product-compliance
Lightning Source LLC
Chambersburg PA
CBHW070104210526
45170CB00012B/739